Biomedical Research:
Collaboration and Conflict of Interest

Biomedical Research: Collaboration and Conflict of Interest

Edited by

Roger J. Porter, M.D.
Deputy Director, National Institute of Neurological Disorders and Stroke
Professor of Neurology and Adjunct Professor of Pharmacology
Uniformed Services University of the Health Sciences
Consultant–Lecturer in Neurology, National Naval Medical Center
Bethesda, Maryland

and

Thomas E. Malone, Ph.D.
Vice President for Biomedical Research
Association of American Medical Colleges
Washington, D.C.

Christopher C. Vaughan
Associate Editor
Bethesda, Maryland

The Johns Hopkins University Press
Baltimore and London

The opinions and assertions contained herein are the private views of the authors and are not to be construed as official or necessarily reflecting the views of the Association of American Medical Colleges, the Office of Science and Technology Policy of the Executive Office of the President, the National Institutes of Health, the United States Public Health Service, the U.S. Department of Health and Human Services, the Uniformed Services University of the Health Sciences, the Department of the Navy or the Naval Service at large, or the U.S. Department of Defense.

The Johns Hopkins University Press
701 West 40th Street
Baltimore, Maryland 21211-2190
The Johns Hopkins Press Ltd., London

 The paper used in this book meets the minimum requirements of the American National Standard for Information Sciences—Permanence of Paper for Printed Library Materials, ANSI Z39.48-1984.

Library of Congress Cataloging-in-Publication Data
Biomedical research : collaboration and conflict of interest / edited by Roger J. Porter and Thomas E. Malone ; Christopher C. Vaughan, associate editor.
   p.   cm.
   Includes bibliographical references and index.
   ISBN 0-8018-4400-2 (alk. paper)
   1. Medicine—Research—United States. 2. Conflict of interests. 3. Universities and colleges—Business management. 4. Industry and education. I. Porter, Roger J., 1942–   . II. Malone, Thomas E., 1926–   . III. Vaughan, Christopher, C, 1961–
   [DNLM: 1. Academic Medical Centers—organization & administration—United States. 2. Ethics. 3. Industry. 4. Research Support—organization & administration—United States. W 20.5 B6155]
   R854.U5B525 1992
   610'.72073—dc20
   DNLM/DLC
for Library of Congress   91–35381
                                                        CIP

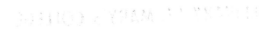

Contents

Foreword

Nearly thirty-five years ago, I began my career as an independent medical investigator. I was assigned a lab by my mentor (and he presumably by our parent university), applied for and was awarded a grant by the National Institutes of Health (NIH), and supplemented this funding with a couple of small grants from industry, ostensibly to perform some drug studies. During that time, most of my salary came from a faculty award supported by a pharmaceutical company. Interpreted in terms of today's ethos, there I was, a fledgling assistant professor, already engaged in an academy-industry relationship. Yet this was not viewed as such either by me or by my industrial sponsors. I viewed their support as simply a means for me to pursue scholarship—that is, to do my research. The award for my salary had been won competitively through the peer-review process, and there was no pressure to do drug-related research even though some of my small grant support was earmarked for that purpose. Some of the grants even came from competing pharmaceutical companies! Terms such as *conflict of interest* had not even been invented, and there was little familiarity with concepts such as patent rights, royalties, intellectual property, venture capital, selective distribution of data, and public disclosure, at least among investigators. The name of the game was knowledge qua knowledge; besides, nobody (of my acquaintance, at least) had enough money to invest in pharmaceutical and biotechnology stocks.

Over the ensuing years, things changed, at first almost imperceptibly. One heard about the investigator who mortgaged his home to buy the stock of a drug company whose drug he was investigating because he thought they had a sure winner and who then made a "killing" on his stocks, or one learned of the occasional laboratory, department, or institution that cut a deal with a drug company or an equipment manufacturer to collaborate on research of mutual interest and benefit. Nobody paid too much attention to these apparently rare occurrences, and nobody thought of them in terms of "conflict." After all, most biomedical research was ultimately aimed at bettering the life of patients, and the industry that aided and abetted this goal was acting in the public good. What was not apparent to most of us was that the culture of the biomedical enterprise was changing from a primary emphasis on scholarship to a focus on entrepreneurial success.

This issue was first called to our attention when Arnold Relman, then editor of the *New England Journal of Medicine,* took to task physicians who had a financial interest in diagnostic facilities to which they referred patients. This practice remains extant, but reimbursement has been outlawed for care rendered to Medicare patients in such facilities. Entrepreneurism in the academy really hit its stride in the 1980s. Major collaborative relationships evolved between industry and medical schools, teaching hospitals, and universities; professors in basic science departments, often armed with privately raised venture capital, started biotechnology companies. Many scientists became consultants to or directors of high-tech firms and not infrequently held equity positions in these firms, and students were often supported by both industry and the university. Serious questions have been raised about clinical investigators owning stock in companies whose therapeutic agents were undergoing clinical trials under their supervision.

These examples are not meant to imply that in any or all of these relationships there were conflicts of interest. On the contrary, in most academic-industrial relationships, conflicts of interest do not exist. Nor should it be inferred that academic-industrial relationships are sinful or harmful or both. What is true is that these relationships, which are examined in detail in this book, may become suspect unless they are carried out in an atmosphere of openness. Equally important, the universities that have faculty members working with industrial products of commercial value must lay down ground rules under which this work is to be carried out. Research performed in the sunshine under clearly specified rules can avoid conflict of interest altogether. As Ralph Waldo Emerson said, "Nothing astonishes men so much as common sense and plain dealing." From where I sit, that is the golden rule that must be applied to academic-industrial relationships.

Robert G. Petersdorf, M.D.
President, Association of American Medical Colleges
Washington, D.C.

Preface

Collaboration between academia and profit-making organizations is by no means new. In fields such as engineering, university departments have long accommodated—even encouraged—funding from industrial sources. One might logically ask, therefore, what is new and different about industrial funding of *biomedical* research, the subject of much current discussion and of this book? The answer lies both in the history of biomedical research and the rapid changes that have taken place in this field, affecting investigators as well as their institutions. This volume provides an analysis of the impact of industry and academia on biomedical research and how these institutions work together. The analysis begins with the moral imperative for biomedical research and ends with an analysis of how the U.S. federal government regulates its own laboratories.

We hope that both policymakers and scientists will benefit from this book. First, we hope to provide insight into the issues for those who govern and those who assist them—the congressional staff. The implications of legislation will, we hope, be seen more clearly in the light of this discussion. Second, we provide a framework for academia and industry in dealing with the multiplicity of potential opportunities and problems in such collaborations. Serving these diverse groups requires careful explanations of complex issues; we hope we have accomplished our task without being overly simplistic.

The book is divided into four parts. The first is introductory; it provides the basics needed to comprehend the importance of medical research. Beginning with the moral imperative (Chapter 1), it progresses to an analysis of funding (Chapter 2) and ends with an analysis of the competitive imperative (Chapter 3).

Part II describes how the academic medical center seeks to gain from its relationship with industry and begins with a brief statement (Chapter 4) of the overall mission of the university and the academic medical center. Once the tone has been set for what the university is all about, Chapter 5 describes the university's point of view regarding collaborative ventures with industry, with emphasis on the problems arising in such ventures and on various solutions to those problems. The last chapter in this section is an extensive review and analysis (chapter 6) of how different academic medical centers are approaching potential opportunities to consummate collaboration with industry.

Part III, looking inward instead of outward, dissects the impact of such collaboration on the academic medical center. First, Chapter 7 begins with a discussion on the nature of scientific observation and of conflicts and then sets forth a thesis about the differing effects on society resulting from conflicts occurring in the basic laboratory, as opposed to those arising in clinical investigation. An analysis of the many forms of personal gain follows (Chapter 8), as it is personal gain—in one way or another—that fuels the fires of conflict of interest. The instrument of conflict of interest in science is observer bias (Chapter 9), without which conflicts would not exist; a full description of the destructive power of observer bias is provided. Finally, the last chapter in this section (Chapter 10) addresses ways to control conflicts of interest—from the most permissive to the most restrictive approaches.

The fourth and final part provides a forum for industry's view of the foregoing issues (Chapter 11) and also for insight into how laboratories operated by the U.S. federal government collaborate with industry (Chapter 12).

Why examine these aspects of biomedical research at this time? First, medical care is becoming extraordinarily expensive, and biomedical research and technology is making a direct contribution to this rapid increase in costs. Second, industry—especially the pharmaceutical industry—has funds to devote to research, thereby making possible research that previously might not be conducted. Third, the potential contribution of biomedical developments to the competitiveness of the United States is not trivial. Fourth, the issues of conflicts of interest have stirred both scientific and political fires. This book addresses these issues and many more.

Acknowledgments

This volume grew from the extraordinary opportunity for one of the editors (RJP) to be a scholar-in-residence in the Division of Biomedical Research of the Association of American Medical Colleges (AAMC), a division that is under the direction of the other editor (TEM). We are therefore grateful to the AAMC—and most especially to its president, Robert G. Petersdorf—for the flexibility and for the collegial academic atmosphere that made this effort possible. Colleagues at the AAMC who were especially generous with their time, either to make informal suggestions or to review outlines and draft chapters, include James Bentley, Donald Kassebaum, Douglas Kelly, Thomas Kennedy, Louis Kettel, Joseph Keyes, Richard Knapp, Elizabeth Martin, Joan Hartman Moore, Herbert Nickens, John Sherman, Edward Stimmler, August Swanson, and Kathleen Turner.

Equally generous in commenting on individual chapters were our colleagues at the National Institute of Neurological Disorders and Stroke (NINDS), including James Dambrosia, Jonas Ellenberg, Marian Emr, Murray Goldstein, Carole Kirby, Pamela Jones, Mary Miers, Richard Sherbert, William Theodore, and Craig Venter. Judy Hallett of the University of Maryland made very constructive comments, as did Albert Teich of the American Association for the Advancement of Science, Michael Gluck of the Office of Technology Assessment, and Carlos Kruytbosch of the National Science Foundation.

Our associate editor, Christopher C. Vaughan of NINDS, was unflaggingly energetic in editing the manuscripts, dealing with the many technical details, and co-authoring a chapter. Elizabeth Garabedian of the National Institutes of Health (NIH) library was very helpful in ferreting out references. Keeping us organized throughout was Susan Free, with the typing assistance of Barbara Bloomquist.

We are most grateful to the Johns Hopkins University Press for publishing the book. Without the persistence, encouragement, and insight of Wendy Harris, this book would not have succeeded.

Finally, we are grateful to the chapter authors. It is, after all, their collective expertise on which we depend.

Contributors

David A. Blake, Ph.D., Senior Associate Dean, The Johns Hopkins University School of Medicine, Baltimore, Maryland

Philip S. Chen, Jr., Ph.D., Associate Director for Intramural Affairs, National Institutes of Health, Bethesda, Maryland

Theodore Cooper, M.D., Ph.D., Chairman of the Board, and Chief Executive Officer, The Upjohn Company, Kalamazoo, Michigan

Alicia K. Dustira, Ph.D., Senior Policy Analyst, Executive Office of the President, Office of Science and Technology Policy, Washington, D.C.

Sheldon Ekland-Olson, Ph.D., Professor, Department of Sociology, University of Texas, Austin, Texas

Thomas E. Malone, Ph.D., Vice President for Biomedical Research, Association of American Medical Colleges, Washington, D.C.

Hans Mark, Ph.D., Chancellor, The University of Texas System, Austin, Texas

Mark Novitch, M.D., Vice Chairman of the Board, The Upjohn Company, Kalamazoo, Michigan

Roger J. Porter, M.D., Deputy Director, National Institute of Neurological Disorders and Stroke, National Institutes of Health, Bethesda, Maryland

Allan C. Shipp, M.H.A., Senior Staff Associate, Division of Biomedical Research, Association of American Medical Colleges, Washington, D.C.

Bruce L. R. Smith, Ph.D., Senior Staff Member, Center for Public Policy Education, The Brookings Institute, Washington, D.C.

Christopher C. Vaughan, B.S., Medical Editor, National Institute of Neurological Disorders and Stroke, National Institutes of Health, Bethesda, Maryland

Paul G. Waugaman, M.P.A., Assistant Vice Chancellor for Research, North Carolina State University, Raleigh, North Carolina

PART I

The Fundamentals of Biomedical Research

1 • The Moral Imperative for Biomedical Research

Thomas E. Malone

Cura ut valeus (Guard your health) was a frequent closing phrase in the days when letters were written in Latin—an attentiveness still reflected in our common casual greeting "How are you?" A concern for health, a natural corollary of the primordial instinct for self-preservation, has been a constant human preoccupation. Yet, until very recently, little real progress was made in understanding the nature of diseases or in evolving effective ways to deal with them. The progress of medicine has, indeed, been tortuous—like groping through a maze on a moonless night.

MEDICINE'S ROCKY ROAD TO MODERNITY

We can assume that ancient civilizations were beset by the same diversity of diseases and conditions that have been prevalent throughout man's existence, notably infectious and parasitic diseases, traumas of all kinds, and skeletal and muscular deteriorations. Man's distinctive capacity for reasoning naturally led him to seek the causes of the ills that beset him: pain, sickness, debility, and death. Where no visible explanations were available, he turned, inevitably, to invisible causes: the supernatural. All ancient and primitive civilizations have created a panoply of gods and demons to whom all inexplicable events, from

I am indebted to Daphne Stamos, for assembling most of the historical material, and especially to George L. Payne, for editing and making substantive contributions to this chapter.

thunderstorms to fevers, could be ascribed. To avert consequent disasters, it thus became necessary to placate angry gods or divert malicious demons. Enter the medicine man, who—with incantations (the precursor of religious liturgy), divination from human or animal sacrifice (the debut of animals in the service of medicine), trickery (the ancestor of both magic and quackery), and the administration of various nostrums (a primitive pharmacology based, in part, on the observed efficacy of some herbs and effusions)—sought to mediate twixt man and the gods.*

All these elements of medical practice have continued to exist, in various forms, throughout history and do so today. Even many clearly irrational superstitions are not yet dead; most of us can empathize with Niels Bohr, the eminent Danish physicist, who, when asked by a visitor whether he believed in the horseshoe hanging on his study wall, replied, "Of course not. But I am told that a horseshoe will bring you good luck whether you believe in it or not."

The vagaries of medical practice have, from time to time, raised shifting moral, political, and theological issues. These must, of course, be seen in the context of their time. Morality is a social code, and contemporaneous values of good and evil will decide what is acceptable ethical behavior at any given time—or what balance of good and evil resulting from an action is regarded as justifiable by society. For example, the ritual sacrifice of a lamb, instead of a firstborn son or a young virgin, became socially acceptable only when it was believed that the substitution was acceptable to the god to whom the sacrifice was offered. It is clearly unreasonable—and, of course, futile—to apply the moral standards of one era to the perceived societal necessities of another. In fact, throughout history, dissent from current practices, beliefs, and precepts has only rarely been tolerated; all too often, it proved hazardous to the critic's health.

In the more advanced civilization of Babylon, circa 2100 B.C., treatment of the sick was in the hands of physician-priests whose ministrations, though still based on ritual and magic, bore the earliest vestiges of traditional medicine. Drugs such as colchicine, opium, and hemp were available. Surgery was practiced but was, of course, performed under septic conditions, without anesthesia. As was to remain true for centuries, very little could be done for an individual with a major disease. Life was short and full of misery—sometimes for the

*Archaeological evidence suggests that Neanderthalers were the first, 50,000 years ago, to have spiritual beliefs. They buried, instead of simply abandoning, their dead and furnished the grave with the physical necessities (food, implements, etc.) needed in an afterlife.

physician who lost his life if a highborn person died as a result of his treatment (the earliest form of a malpractice judgment) (Woodward 1989).

Eventually, it was the philosophers, particularly in Greece and Egypt, who sought to base their speculative attempts at a more rational explanation of disease on observations and anatomical investigations. However, without even the vestige of a coherent scientific base, their theories, more often than not, still had religious and mythical foundations. The boundaries separating science, religion, and the supernatural were indistinct, and their intertwining provided little support for interpreting the mysteries of the world, including the human condition.

Celsus (in *De medicina,* circa A.D. 30) noted that it was Hippocrates (who flourished circa 460 B.C.) "who first separated medicine from philosophy" by insisting on careful observation, untrammeled by preconceived ideas, as the basis for teaching medicine. Hippocrates is, indeed, revered as the "Father of Medicine," though the 100 or so medical works now known as the "Hippocratic Collection" had many authors over a period of some 800 years (from the fifth century B.C. to the third century A.D.). What is noteworthy, as Charles Singer (*Encyclopedia Britannica,* 14th ed.) pointed out, is that "the works of the Collection contain nothing of superstition. They are sometimes wearisomely sophistic; they are frequently ludicrously wrong; they often advance absurd hypotheses; they are not seldom obscure. But the attitude of their authors to the supernatural is the same throughout and none swerves in his loyalty to the idea of 'natural law.'"

Hippocrates is now best remembered for defining a standard of conduct for physicians in what is known as the "Hippocratic Oath," which is still a part of the graduating ceremonies at most medical schools—even though it is only loosely observed. In the first part of the oath, dealing with the propagation of the medical profession, the fledgling physician, for example, promises to share his substance with his teachers, to support him, if he be in need, and to teach his children, if they desire it, "without fee or covenant." He also undertakes to "impart this Art by precept, by lecture and by every mode of teaching," to his own sons and to "disciples bound by covenant and oath, according to the Law of Medicine." The second part, dealing with his duties toward his patients, opens with the oft-quoted sentence: "The regimen I adopt shall be for the benefit of my patients according to my ability and judgment, and not for their hurt or for any wrong." It continues,

> I will give no deadly drug to any, though it be asked of me, nor will I counsel such, and especially I will not aid a woman to procure abortion.

Whatsoever house I enter, there will I go for the benefit of the sick, refraining from all wrongdoing or corruption, and especially from any act of seduction, of male or female, of bond or free. Whatsoever things I see or hear concerning the life of men, in my attendance on the sick or even apart therefrom, which ought not to be noised abroad, I will keep silence thereon, counting such things to be as sacred secrets. (*Encyclopedia Britannica,* 15th ed., 1974)

Even though the scientific content of medicine was hardly even rudimentary, the ethical context of the practice of medicine and of the conduct of the physician was already clearly perceived.

Among the Greeks, Galen (Major 1954) stands out as advocating what we would call the "scientific method": the use of rational and understandable methods to search for objective explanations of events. Galen insisted that every theoretical conclusion must be proven by experiment. He studied medicine for eleven years, circa A.D. 115, in Alexandria, then the center of the Greek world. Disappointed by the scant knowledge of his teachers, he codified medical terminology in forty-five books, studied wounds and injuries of gladiators, and carried out investigations in anatomy and physiology on humans, apes, hogs, and other animals. He wrote more than twelve volumes, a thousand pages each, setting forth what was to be basic medical knowledge (not all correct) for the next fifteen centuries. Indeed, Galen was required reading for medical students at Oxford University until the beginning of this century.

The rational approach to medical problems that had now evolved, of course, relieved both gods and demons of responsibility for man's ills—but only temporarily.

What might have been a steady progress in the evolution of scientific medical knowledge was interrupted by the so-called bubonic plague of Justinian, which ravaged Europe for fifty years (A.D. 540–590); some cities were completely depopulated, and it is estimated that 100 million people died (somewhere between two thirds and three quarters of the population). This catastrophe destroyed all faith in the accumulated learning of Greek and Roman medicine, which had been powerless to stop or even alleviate the disaster. For the next thousand years, little, if anything, was added to recorded medical knowledge. Learning was virtually confined to the rapidly growing Christian Church, which now held that pestilence and disease were divine retribution for men's sins. The Church did, however, minister to the sick, and it preserved in its monasteries, during the long Dark Ages, the Greek and Latin medical manuscripts.

The revival of interest in Greek and Roman culture, which launched the Renaissance in the thirteenth century, also brought a fresh outlook and new intellectual energy to virtually all fields of endeavor. The first medical school in Europe, at Salerno, Italy, was given a virtual monopoly on medical teaching in 1221 by the Holy Roman Emperor. The universities that were established—Bologna (chartered 1158), Paris (chartered 1201), Oxford (four colleges founded between 1249 and 1278), Cambridge (1284)—had their roots in monasteries, long the sole repository of literacy. However, while theology was their primary focus, law and medicine were included in their curricula. The first independent medical school in England, St. Thomas's Hospital Medical School in London, also dates from the thirteenth century. Instruction, however, was confined to the traditional texts.

The turning of the calendar from 1299 to 1300 had a profound psychological effect. The new century was regarded as a new opportunity and challenge. Man's innate curiosity and inventiveness, muffled and dormant during the Dark Ages, began to reassert themselves. Medical research slowly came back to life.

Unlike the sixth-century bubonic plague, the "Black Death" (its pneumonic form whose hemorrhages turn the skin dark), that ravaged Asia and Europe from 1346 to 1361 and killed more than a third of the population, did not tarnish the reputation of the medical profession. The Church stuck to its theological guns and interpreted the plague as God's punishment for man's sins and a stern reminder of His existence. To assuage the divine wrath, Pope Clement VI declared 1348 a Holy Year and invited Christians to make a pilgrimage to Rome. More than 1,250,000 responded, which merely served to spread the infection, and only 10 percent survived this pilgrimage. There was, however, a clue to a more rational explanation for the pandemic in the observation that coughing and sneezing spread the disease, and people were ruthless in abandoning those, including family members, who did (Panati 1989). Eventually, it was decided that the plague was caused by poison put into the wells by the Jews. Although the Pope formally exonerated the Jews, the persecutions continued; some ruling nobles were only too glad to have an excuse for getting rid of their creditors.

In 1543, Andreas Vesalius published a new book on anatomy that corrected many of Galen's errors. Enthusiasm for scientific research began to blossom in the 1600s, and the seeds were sown for the growth of modern scientific knowledge (Bloch 1987). Their slow germination is a measure—and an inescapable function—of the complexity of the matters with which the medical sciences must deal.

Meanwhile, living conditions remained grim. Life expectancy is estimated to have been between twenty and forty years (Covey 1989). Mortality from infection (including endemic pestilences), childbirth, hemorrhage, and other diseases and ailments was very high. Increased population pressure, poor housing and sanitation, rodent infestation, and polluted water contributed to the rapid spread of diseases such as smallpox, typhus, dysentery, and syphilis, which often wiped out masses of people. The last and mildest of the great plagues—the bubonic plague in London from May to December of 1665—resulted in the death of almost 70,000 of the city's 400,000 population. In fact, the chances of living a long and healthy life were so slim that longevity was often viewed as an undesirable extension of one's vulnerability to pain and suffering. Aging was regarded as a symptom of bodily decay and a sign of human failure and an undesirable alternative to an earlier death (Covey 1989). And the Church, of course, held out the appealing prospect of a trouble-free sojourn in eternity.

The importance of health was a common theme of writers and politicians, and there was clear recognition of the societal imperative of medical research. For example, Michel de Montaigne, French courtier and essayist, wrote that "health is a precious thing, and the only one, in truth, which deserves that we employ in its pursuit not only time, sweat, trouble, and worldly goods, but even life; As far as I am concerned, no road that would lead us to health is either arduous or expensive." In England, Thomas Dekker and John Webster put it more succinctly in their play *Westward Hoe* (1604): "Gold that buys health can never be ill spent." Philosopher-mathematician Rene Descartes, thirteen years before his death, expressed an apparently unfulfilled resolve "to devote what time I may still have to live to no other occupation than of endeavoring to acquire some knowledge of Nature, which shall be of such a kind as to enable us therefrom to deduce rules in Medicine of greater certainty than those at present in use."

Major scientific contributions of the time were made by Francis Bacon and William Harvey. Bacon was a lawyer, politician, and judge whose writings defined scientific methods. He emphasized structured experiments with careful control factors and conclusions drawn from evidence. In 1628, William Harvey published *Exercitatio Anatomica de Motu Cordis et Sanguinis in Animalibus,* in which he described the circulation of blood—a momentous step toward the understanding of bodily functions.

Pharmacology during this era was limited, but the use of wine as a therapeutic agent was universally accepted. Ambroise Pare, late in the sixteenth century, used wine as an ointment base to save injured soldiers from wound suppuration that led to sepsis, gangrene, or tetanus; theretofore, many had died because suppuration was thought to be a healthy, curative process. The first *London Pharmacopoeia* was published in 1618 and recommended medicated wine as an appetite stimulant, diuretic, sedative, and overall contributor to states of physical and emotional well-being. We can still drink to that.

Medical practice was, however, benignly vicious. Dominated by belief in "the four humours," the treatments of choice were bloodletting, emetics, purgatives, enemas (known as "clysters"), and irritation of the nasal cavity to induce sneezing—all designed to restore the balance of the body fluids, whose imbalance was thought to cause disease. The draconian treatment of England's Charles II, who apparently suffered a stroke in 1685, is chronicled in the diary of his chief physician: seven bloodlettings; three enemas; two emetics; three purgatives; a nose irritation; a plaster of Spanish fly, mustard, and camphor on his shaved head; and four pharmaceuticals—quinine; extract of human skull; a concoction of flowers, pearls, and sugar; and, finally, an extract of all the herbs and animals in the kingdom. The king, who had regained consciousness several times during this ordeal, died on the sixth day, quite probably as a result of the treatment he received (Panati 1989).

Bloodletting, by incision or by leeches, persisted until the late 1800s. Clysters were popular as preventive medicine; in France, Louis XIV (d. 1715) and important members of his court had as many as four a day. They were superseded, with the development of antisepsis, by surgical removal of the colon, which continued in England and the United States, as an elective prophylaxis, until the 1930s, when it was replaced by "colonic irrigation" (alias clyster), then by the regular use of laxatives, and now, of course, by high-fiber diets.

In fact, until the beginning of this century, a patient who did not receive treatment seems to have had a considerably better chance of recovery than a similar patient who did. Only then were some physicians enlightened, and honest, enough to have doubts about the efficacy of their stock in trade. Dr. Oliver Wendell Holmes (d. 1894) wrote, "I firmly believe that if the whole materia medica, as now used, could be sunk to the bottom of the sea, it would be all the better for mankind—and all the worse for the fishes," a sentiment more recently echoed by Dr. Martin Fishbein (d. 1962) who, however, said that only "half the modern drugs could well be thrown out the window, except that the birds might eat them." It is estimated that somewhere between 1910 and 1912, a random patient in this country, with a random disease, consulting a doctor chosen at random had, for the first time in the history of mankind, a better than fifty:fifty chance of profiting from the encounter (Henderson 1964).

The development of histology, at the end of the eighteenth century, is attributed to the Frenchman Xavior Bichat (Breo 1990) whose research led to the identification of twenty-one body tissues such as arterial, muscular, and nervous. His work paved the way for the study of pathology in the nineteenth century by Koch and Virschow, the latter having finally dispelled the theory of spontaneous generation.

Controversy over *germ theory* (every living thing must have a parent) versus spontaneous generation started in antiquity and continued sporadically through the ages. Although Anton von Leeuwenhoek (1632–1720) was the first to see and describe bacteria, during the early development of microscopes, their role in disease was not recognized until the late 1800s, when Louis Pasteur, by proving the bacterial origin of fermentation, set the stage for Joseph Lister's introduction of antiseptic surgery and Robert Koch's discovery of the tuberculosis bacillus in 1882. These developments launched the new science of bacteriology, which opened the door for the conquest of infectious diseases.

Another major technological advance during the 1800s was Rene Laennec's invention (c. 1819) of the stethoscope, which greatly facilitated the study of cardiology and the diagnosis of respiratory ailments.

The beginning of the twentieth century has been called the age of "descriptive medicine." Advances in microscopy and bacteriology helped physicians to establish causal relationships of illness and to understand the process of infection; however, although doctors could recognize and diagnose illness, medicine was often ineffective in its abilities to treat infections and other afflictions. Average life expectancy in 1900 in Massachusetts was 46.1 years for males and 49.4 years for females. For those who survived childhood, life expectancy was much greater: An average man of 20 could expect to live to be 61.8 years old, and a woman could expect to live to be 63.7. This discrepancy suggests that infant and child mortality rates were high, and indeed the infant mortality rate in Massachusetts in 1900 was 141.1 per 1000 live births (Wattenberg and the U.S. Bureau of the Census 1970). Children had to run the gauntlet of childhood diseases, which struck indiscriminately and unrelentingly. Common killers of the day included tuberculosis, typhoid fever, scarlet fever and streptococcal throat infection, diphtheria, whooping cough, diabetes mellitus, cardiovascular-renal disease, influenza and pneumonia, gastrointestinal disorders, and accidents.

However, scientific progress resulted in improved diagnostic and therapeutic techniques. Surgery was revolutionized by Joseph Lister's concept of germ-free environments through the use of carbolic acid spray. The use of anesthesia permitted more lengthy and sophisticated procedures. Surgical intervention offered hope to those with breast and cervical cancer and some forms of stomach cancer. The first radical mastectomy was performed in 1891 by William Halsted at Johns Hopkins and served to exemplify options offered by surgery to those suffering from cancer. Wilhelm Roentgen's discovery of x-rays, in 1895, created a powerful new diagnostic tool, and the use of radium in radiotherapy offered a hopeful option for cancer patients.

The first major biomedical advance in our century was the production of antibiotics. For the first time in history, bacterial infections could actually be stopped. Penicillin, derived from the mold *Penicillium* in 1941 in Britain, became available by 1944 for widespread use in the treatment of infected American and British soldiers during World War II, thus saving many lives that would have been lost without it. More sophisticated antibiotics developed over the next fifty years have provided effective treatments for almost every bacterial infection. Once intractable diseases (such as syphilis, streptococcal infections and their sequelae, and bacterial pneumonia) are no longer major killers. Nevertheless, the changing nature of bacterial threats (due to selective replications and mutations that create hardy strains) obviously demands that antibiotic research be kept current.

By the mid-1950s, vaccinations were effective in protecting children against traditional childhood killers such as whooping cough, tetanus, diphtheria, measles, and rubella. A dramatic achievement was the vaccination against poliomyelitis, a disease which, in the early 1950s, caused some 25,000 cases of paralysis each year and sentenced many young people to death or to life in an iron lung. Another triumph of medical technology was vaccination against smallpox, which resulted in the worldwide eradication of a much-feared infectious disease that had caused disfigurement and death for centuries. It is estimated that in the eighteenth century, up to 20 percent of all deaths were due to smallpox.

The impact that biomedical research has already had on the quality of life is impressive. In the United States, by 1988, estimates of life expectancy at birth were 71.8 years for males and 78.6 years for females; an individual surviving to 20 could expect to live another 61.0 years, for a total life expectancy of 81 years. In 1988, the birth mortality rate was at an all-time low at 10.1 per 1000 live births, a 1400 percent improvement from 1900! These statistics (U.S. Department of Health and Human Services 1992) illustrate the benefits of the application of new knowledge through more effective medical intervention and through wider and better public health measures (improved sanitation, clean drinking water, and other steps to inhibit the spread of infection).

During the second half of the twentieth century, there has been a scientific revolution of unparalleled scope and intensity. It has been said, without exaggeration, that biomedicine has now joined nuclear physics and space technology as the third "big science." The developments that have brought this about can fairly be called "an explosion of knowledge."

AN EXPLOSION OF KNOWLEDGE

Just as the emergence of bacteriology had opened the doors to the conquest of infectious diseases at the beginning of this century, so the maturation of genetic research showed the way to dealing with congenital diseases, disabilities, and predispositions to disease in midcentury. The first research on inheritance was done by Gregor Mendel, who published his conclusions in 1865, but little further happened until his work was rediscovered in 1900. The study of DNA (deoxyribonucleic acid), the carrier of the genetic code, began in the 1930s at the Rockefeller Institute. In 1953, Watson and Crick, at Cambridge University, published the results of their research, which postulated that DNA was a double-stranded pyrimidine and purine base-pair system, popularized as "the double helix." Their work, for which they won a Nobel prize in 1962, triggered an explosion of research in molecular biology. By the end of the 1950s, approximately a dozen single-gene defects were identified as causing enzyme-deficiency diseases. The structure of DNA, its replication, transcription, translation, and other mysteries of the genetic code were rapidly revealed. By 1980, over 1000 genetic disorders were identified (such as glycogen storage disorders, hemophilia and thalassemia, alkaptonuria, and albinism, to name a few), which made possible prenatal screening and conclusive diagnostic methods.

Recombinant-DNA techniques have resulted in many useful applications, including methods for genetic and viral testing, a safe hepatitis B vaccine, and myriad laboratory investigative capabilities. The understanding of the process of active immunization, vaccination, and drug resistance, and the creation of pure antigens and antibodies through these techniques promise to relieve thousands of potential victims from maladies such as malaria, now the world's number one killer, and Chagas's disease, the scourge of South America. The study of the major histocompatibility complex will improve the success of organ transplantation and promises to explain why some individuals have adverse reactions to vaccines.

The Human Genome Project is a plan to map the function and structure of the entire human genome, some 100,000 genes, within twenty years. Through recombinant-DNA methods, scientists have recently isolated or approximated the location of genes associated with juvenile diabetes, melanoma, rheumatoid arthritis, and retinitis pigmentosa. The gene responsible for cystic fibrosis was identified in the summer of 1989 after a twenty-year effort, and today, by identifying affected fetuses in utero, treatment programs can begin at birth, with the prospects of much better results. The potential uses of this knowledge of the human genome range from the ability to screen for inborn disorders to the use of genetic engineering techniques to repair malfunctioning cellular DNA.

Research has now brought us face to face with a tempting but potentially dangerous challenge: the ability to select or alter a person's genetic composition.

The applications of the genome project and recombinant-DNA techniques will also provide the medical community with a powerful weapon against some chronic illnesses and against such major threats as the current human immunodeficiency virus (HIV) epidemic. The power of this new resource is illustrated by the rapid progress in understanding HIV itself. In less than ten years—a remarkably short time for such a complex endeavor—biomedical researchers have identified this virus and have studied its replication cycle, mode of infection, and genetic makeup, and there is good reason to expect that effective intervention will follow. Meanwhile, publicity for what is already known about HIV has substituted hope for despair and has helped to inhibit, though it cannot quite dispel, the latent tendency to see a supernatural origin for such a scourge. Though it may appear to be a curious contradiction, a predilection for blaming and then seeking the aid of the gods is an irrational product of man's ability to reason. In former times, this new epidemic, with a slow course of progression and an apparent 100 percent fatality rate, would have been as disastrous as the plagues; it would inexorably have ravaged populations with attendant public hysteria and the disruption of normal activities.

The power of genetic research to mitigate the effects of this epidemic and eventually to bring it under control must weigh heavily in the balance against the apprehensions about possible misuses of the new techniques.

Gene therapy offers the possibility of treating hundreds, even thousands, of disorders that were heretofore incurable. A glimpse of this extraordinary potential has been provided by research conducted just since September 1990, when W. French Anderson and his colleagues at NIH initiated the first federally approved use of human gene therapy. A 4-year-old girl was given gene therapy for a rare disorder resulting in severe immunodeficiency, characterized by depletion of all T lymphocytes (white blood cells). This deficiency manifests itself clinically as an extreme and fatal susceptibility to a wide range of infections. It is due to the inheritance of two copies of a gene that normally encodes for an enzyme known as adenosine deaminase (ADA). The normal ADA gene was inserted into billions of the young patient's T cells and then reinfused into her blood. By April of 1991, the patient had normal levels of circulating lymphocytes and of some antibodies, indicating that, thus far, her immune system had returned to normal.

Another team at NIH, led by Steven Rosenberg, has demonstrated the potential for gene therapy in the treatment of cancer. Rosenberg's strategy is based on the discovery of a naturally occurring substance in the body, known as tumor necrosis factor (TNF), which actually shrinks tumors. Lymphocytes were removed from several patients with melanoma and were exposed to viruses that carry the gene for TNF. This gene is incorporated into the DNA of the lymphocytes, which are then grown in large quantities and reinjected into the blood stream of the cancer patients. It is expected that these activated lymphocytes will seek out the tumor, attack the cancerous cells, and release TNF to finish them off.

A variety of other diseases and disorders are being examined actively for their susceptibility to treatment through gene therapy. These include cystic fibrosis, breast cancer, colon cancer, emphysema, molecular abnormalities associated with the fragile-X syndrome, and others. At the same time, carriers other than retroviruses are being considered for gene insertion into internal organs, blood vessels, and young embryos. The promise of gene therapy should be greatly enhanced by the Human Genome Project, making it possible to envision a time when physicians will be able routinely to treat genetic disorders caused not only by single defective genes but also by complexes of genes.

Realistic hope is being offered by the prospect of inserting genetically engineered cells to produce clotting factors for hemophiliacs, insulin-producing cells for diabetics, and dopamine-producing cells for the neurons in the brains of those with Parkinson's disease. Similar approaches offer potential help for AIDS through the use of constructed cells that will produce soluble CD-4, the receptors found on immune cells that are attacked by HIV. It is hoped that the engineered receptors will act as decoys and bind the HIV so that immune cells will not be attacked in as high concentrations. Further research will give better insight into hyperlipidemia disorders, control of hypertension, causes and management of obesity, biochemical pathways of the brain, peripheral and central nerve regeneration, and many other medical problems.

With so much already accomplished and so much more to be expected from research on this new biomedical frontier, its continued support and, indeed, further stimulation are clear societal imperatives. Yet some potential uses of a technique that, essentially, manipulates heredity raises fears that cast doubt on its morality. The danger, however, lies not in the technique but in the purposes for which it is used, and that is in the hands of those who employ it or, more worrisomely, in those who control or direct its employment. In a world in which ethnic, racial, and religious rivalries regularly overwhelm tolerance and decency—even to the point of flouting self-interest—and in which tyrants are not merely tolerated but extolled as defenders of some delusory faith, the potential for evil applications of good works is ever-present. This concern, of course, is not unique to genetic manipulation; it is equally true of the other two areas of "big science," atomic energy and space technology, to whose existence we have somehow already become more or less reconciled. As bioengineering will undoubtedly bring more benefit to more people more quickly than either of its big-science siblings, there is a compelling moral imperative for its vigorous pursuit.

The other major area in the life sciences that is making rapid and impressive progress is instrumentation. The products created by chemists, physicists, and engineers (such as magnetic resonance imaging (MRI), sonotopography, computed axial tomography (CAT) scanning, cell-culture techniques, and others) have greatly enhanced the experimental, diagnostic, and therapeutic approaches available to today's scientific and medical community. The field of biotechnology has grown enormously in recent years and has become one of the most dynamic sectors of American industry. The expansion and flourishing of this business has played a part in stimulating the economy; investments in the area have yielded dividends several times greater than their principal, and the humanitarian benefits have been incalculable.

The economic impact of biomedical research is greatest—though less readily documented—in the costs and losses that do not occur because illness was prevented, ameliorated, or rapidly cured. The polio vaccine, for example, saved millions of dollars both in the treatment of those who would have contracted it and in the aftercare of those who would have been crippled by this disease. In a modern epidemic, such as AIDS, the cost of treatment and care of victims and the accompanying loss of productivity could become a devastating financial drain if the virus were to continue to spread without cure or effective management. Crass fiscal prudence dictates an economic imperative for biomedical research.

The tremendous technology that now serves the practice of medicine is, of course, a natural progression from the past efforts—the triumphs and failures—of the researchers and practitioners who, brick by brick, built the impressive scientific edifice we inhabit today. During this century, the pace of progress has steadily accelerated and has now reached an almost frightening speed. It is the rapidity of change, as well as the nature of the newest developments, that give rise to concerns about where science is taking us. No one would have predicted, even fifty years ago, that before the year 2000 we would be able to tailor our heredity (while we wreck our environment) or put a man on the moon. Obviously, we cannot predict what the next century will bring. The prospect of living a long life, free from inherited or acquired disabilities, which the biomedical sciences seem to make attainable, may be no better than the prospect of succumbing to the pressures of an overpopulated world with an increasingly hostile environment inimical to life as we know it, which the politico-economic establishment seems to make inevitable. The choice may still be ours, if we can agree, before it is too late, that the only really vital moral imperative is to redress the planet's man-made disabilities and keep it a safe habitat for its varied forms of life.

While our decisions on other moral questions will matter little if we let the environmental question go by default, we are inevitably involved in often-heated debate over the impact of science on society and the extent to which its capabilities should be given free reign. There are also more specific ethical issues, such as the management of population overgrowth (which might be expected to accompany the prolongation of life) and the social ramifications of dealing with those who are not genetically "perfect."

Thomas Jefferson, in a letter to a friend (dated August 10, 1787), wrote, "Health is the first requisite after morality." Because he was actively interested in science and in the advancement of knowledge, one may wonder whether he would, today, be among those who fear that future efforts to reduce morbidity and mortality will also bring about a loss of morality.

THE THORNS ON THE ROSES

Cost-benefit analysis is a common tool for deciding whether support for a given area of research or its application should be increased, continued, or diminished and, often (as, for example, in Medicare and Medicaid), with what restrictions or rules. It is, at best, a rough-and-ready guide: costs are usually underestimated, and benefits—being, in any case, not wholly predictable—are exaggerated. Despite the imperfection, it is, however, proper and prudent to weigh the evil of cost against the good of benefit in assessing the economic imperatives.

The analogy holds for assessing the moral imperatives of biomedical research and its applications. But weighing the foreseen benefits of medical interventions, research procedures, and policies against their real or suspected risks of doing harm is a much more difficult task than deciding levels of support. As the nature and extent of both the good and the evil are usually only based on expectations, rather than knowledge, the debate tends to be highly subjective and, all too often, purely emotional—especially if the objections are not about physical risks but about alleged impropriety (e.g., invasion of privacy), religious tenets, or plain prejudice.

Nor do the benefits and risks remain constant. What may have been a tenable assessment at one time may subsequently prove to be patently wrong. Vaccination against smallpox is a case in point. When Edward Jenner introduced vaccination against the smallpox virus (in 1796, a hundred years before the existence of viruses was even discovered), he made possible the virtual eradication of a major cause of death. Vaccination was clearly a moral imperative and the vaccination of children became an almost universal practice. Even when the virus had been almost eliminated, vaccinations were continued as a wise precaution against its resurgence. In fact, the United States required all immigrants and citizens returning from abroad to have evidence of a successful smallpox vaccination until the early 1970s, when the requirement was withdrawn because the British government announced that it would no longer permit smallpox vaccination. The British had, in effect, decided on a new moral imperative. The fact (at first unobserved and later simply accepted) that smallpox vaccination of children sometimes, though rarely, resulted in mental retardation now outweighed the risk of a smallpox infection. The moral debate was aptly illustrated by two U.S. Public Health Service physicians: When one of them argued that, because the virus still existed, especially in Africa, and the cases of mental retardation were so few, continued vaccination was still the greatest good for the greatest number, a colleague replied, "Would you like to explain that to the parents of a child you have just retarded?"

A serious and urgent moral question is posed by the unprecedentedly rapid population growth brought about by our growing ability and willingness to interfere with nature's ruthless but effective measures for population control: high infant mortality; high childbirth mortality, restricting the population source; a large palette of diseases to shorten the life span; and periodic pandemics to make room for renewed population growth. Starvation due to crop failures and deaths from disasters (such as the recurring typhoons in Bangladesh) have not yet been curbed by man's ingenuity—and may, in fact, have increased due to disregard for the environment. On the other hand, we have developed, and periodically see fit to use, ever-more-effective tools for mass destruction; we countenance political upheavals that send masses scurrying to unsanitary refugee camps that increase the death rate, especially among children; and some governments blatantly engage in genocide. We must assume, however, that, on balance, the world population will continue its rapid increase.

The prospect of an ever-larger population with an ever-growing elderly component raises such mundane questions as whether we can financially support a large number of, say, 100-year olds who may have been retired for 35 years. More serious problems will arise in providing for sufficient sources of food, adequate waste and pollution management, increased demand for energy, and, eventually, simply *lebensraum*. There are reasons to question whether the planet was designed to accommodate and sustain the expected superpopulation even if we were not rapidly limiting its inhabitability by the environmental abuse it has had to endure since the start of the Industrial Revolution.

While it is probably not enough to look to the scientific community, which brought about the Industrial Revolution, for solutions to the problems it has created, efforts in this direction must be on the agenda. For example, the production of nutritionally perfect foodstuffs through bioengineering techniques may help to avert shortages in the food supply or at least fill in links of a broken food chain. Medicine and pharmacology should provide solutions to problems associated with aging and for diseases associated with the environment, such as some melanomas, and lung and liver disorders. Space exploration may provide an understanding of the dynamics of the atmosphere that might lead to remedies for pollution and the repair of the ozone layer or even provide a gateway to new territory to colonize—an idea no crazier now than the prospect of walking on the moon was a century ago.

A more immediate solution, however, lies in a better understanding of the biochemical nature of reproduction that will lead to improved techniques of birth control and their mandatory adoption, throughout the world, to limit population growth—a tactic that only China is already seeking to employ.

Another important ethical problem lies in the social implications of the availability of genetic testing and the use of gene therapy. If access to such diagnostic and therapeutic methods is, in effect, limited to a select population or social class—as might result from some proposed restrictions (such as those on abortion)—will the individual suffering from a genetic handicap bear the brunt not only of disability but also of social discrimination? We must consider whether the presence of such a handicap should be allowed to limit social mobility, whether employers and insurance companies will have access to such information and be tempted to discriminate against those less than genetically perfect, and whether the applications of gene therapy will create additional racial tension if the benefits of the technology are not widespread and available to everyone.

There are more disturbing questions. Is abortion a humane or even tolerable course for fetuses that exhibit genes for serious congenital diseases or for genetic vulnerability to later onset of incurable debilitating diseases? Must genetic testing to select babies of a desired sex, eye color, or hair color be prevented? Many people believe that the emerging techniques are sufficiently subject to abuse that their use must be stringently regulated and closely monitored and controlled.

The possibility of altering an individual's genetic composition or DNA blueprint is a fascinating prospect with both alluring and chilling implications. It remains to be seen whether changing the genome of somatic (i.e., nonreproductive) cells could have severe consequences or side effects—and, if so, how they could be managed—or if treatment for a non-life-threatening problem might even have an unforeseen fatal outcome. If germ cells (which affect inheritance) are involved, progeny will also carry the changed DNA; thus, not only would the patient be treated for a defect, but so would his or her future offspring. Will such changes in the genetic pool have a significant impact on evolution, or are they merely an additional factor in the process of natural selection?

These questions come perilously close to a subject that is seldom openly discussed, but that should be of serious concern: the degradation of human genetic inheritance resulting from medicine's ability and society's apparent demand to save and bring to reproductive age persons who are physically and mentally disadvantaged—many of whom nature, unattended, would have allowed to die before reproducing. For sentimental and humanitarian reasons, none of what has been learned about animal husbandry and effective breeding practices has been applied to human reproduction. This is understandable and perhaps inevitable, but it is nonetheless disturbing that humans have devoted so much skill and effort to exploiting the gene pool of domestic animals and willfully neglected their own. Even the animals in the wild, through survival of the fittest and fierce competition in the mating game, have a better genetic inheritance.

There have been a few attempts to pursue a sterner course. The Spartans, who were famous for their stamina and physique, bathed their newborns in an icy mountain stream and killed all babies that were deformed. (Some primitive peoples are said to have killed excess female infants, but their motives seem to have been economic: fewer mouths to feed now and hereafter.) Now, to take advantage of genetic engineering to repair our own damaged gene pool would seem to be at least as important as, and much more possible than, repairing the hole in the ozone layer. If the techniques that are rapidly becoming available were fully exploited, it might be expected that in future generations everyone will have reached the age-old goal of *mens sana in corpore sano*.

SCIENCE, MORALITY, AND ANIMALS

Animals have been an indispensable tool—one is tempted to say *partner,* but *tool* is more accurate—in biomedical research. Their role has been critical to almost every medical achievement. A biomedical research establishment without animals would be like an army without infantry, and it may as well be admitted that animals are sometimes the cannon fodder in the battle against disease. People who patriotically cheer on soldiers to political wars should be equally grateful to those who bear the brunt of the medical wars. In fact, however, the moral legitimacy of using animals in research has become a vociferously debated public issue.

While ethical considerations date back to antiquity, when research on animals played a major role in freeing medicine from the miasma of superstitious dogma, the present furor is of unprecedented prominence and vehemence. The segment of society that questions the use of animals in research has grown to a large and powerful coalition that ranges from groups who have the traditional concerns for the welfare of animals to those who maintain that any use of animals reflects bias favoring our own species and is therefore immoral. The animal welfare organizations that have existed since the nineteenth century seek primarily to avoid unnecessary suffering and to demand better treatment for and more strictly regulated use of laboratory animals. The new recruits to the cause, however, oppose what is now called "speciesism"—analogous to racism and sexism—and demand equal treatment for animals. It is not always clear whether they intend that medical experimentation should be confined to human subjects or whether animal and human subjects should share the burden equally. In practice, they seem to think that all medical experimentation is wrong. How medicine can advance without experimentation is, of course, not their problem.

A pragmatic justification for the use of animals in research can be derived from a consideration of the evolutionary process—a process that has not only produced the great diversity of species but has also resulted in the disappearance of those that did not meet the challenge of environmental changes. The exigencies of survival dominate the life of each species. The stronger or more intelligent species remain extant by preying on species lower in the food chain. In nature, daily life is a precarious balance between hunting and being hunted (except that herbivores need only worry about the latter). In a strictly evolutionary sense, it can be said that each species survives in accordance with its genetic adaptation and advantage. The Judeo-Christian tradition is that man stands at the pinnacle of the evolutionary tree and was ordained to "have dominion over the fish of the sea, and over the fowl of the air, and over every living thing that moveth upon the earth" (Genesis 1:28).

Nonetheless, the dogma that lower forms of life were created for the indiscriminate use of mankind, though still embraced by some, is no longer tenable for the majority of rational thinkers. Despite the atavistic behavior in some members of society, we do have a brain "with a neocortex capable of verbal communications, projective and abstract logic, and other attributes not found in lower animals" (Vischer 1975). Human beings need not yield solely to instinctive behavior but can control their actions in rational ways that could, and should, include ethical concerns for the mutual welfare of all inhabitants of the earth. These concerns do not deny the use of animals for survival or for the enhancement of the quality of life for present and future generations. Indeed, the central challenge to man today is to continue to improve the human condition and to survive in a healthy state on a planet that makes this goal increasingly difficult. The moral question has to take account of the value of animal research in the alleviation of disease within a framework of laws and policies that ensure humane treatment of the animals.

The trouble with the dogma of dominion over all living things, humanely executed or not, is that it fails to account for the creatures that really stand at the pinnacle of the food chain: the bacteria and the viruses that feed on man and beast alike. The principal role of medicine is to protect us from these myriad predators who are ever-ready to do us in but over whom the Creator failed to give us ex cathedra dominion. Nor should it be thought reprehensible to have the animals, who are equally at risk, join forces with us and, to the best of their limited abilities, contribute to the common good. Biomedical research benefits animals as well as humans: A veterinarian is as likely to prescribe an antibiotic for your cat as your physician is for you.

It cannot be emphasized too strongly that virtually all the most important medical advances have involved animal experimentation and would have been impossible without it. The greatest challenges still lie ahead. Effective defenses must yet be found for a monotonous catalogue of rampant diseases: cancer, heart disease, diabetes, many viral infections, AIDS, Alzheimer's and Parkinson's diseases, rheumatoid arthritis and other autoimmune diseases, cystic fibrosis, dementias, pain, sickle cell disease, and spinal cord injury, to name only the most obvious.

On the question of the moral imperative of using animals in research, the answer of the scientist and of those who have benefited, or hope to benefit, from research must be that it would be immoral not to seek and to use the fruit of such research to diminish or eradicate disease and to improve the quality of life. If this moral imperative had been denied a century or two ago, the present state of health care would be too horrendous for contemporary society to contemplate. A visit to the doctor's quarters on "Old Ironsides," the USS *Constitution* in Boston harbor, would serve as a vivid reminder. Records kept by the physician reveal that in the case of an infected leg that had become gangrenous, amputation was the only alternative for saving a sailor's life. Without antibiotics, general anesthesia, or aseptic techniques, a patient would be given an extra portion of rum and the doctor would saw away. The average time for an amputation was 1 minute 32 seconds (the record was a little over 30 seconds) of excruciating pain, followed by a lifetime of disability.

No sane person would want to turn back the clock to such a procedure, to the ravages of polio, diphtheria, smallpox, or cholera, and to a life expectancy of 30 years. Yet there are those who would now stop the clock and deny future generations the benefits of the even more dramatic advances that obviously lie ahead—who would, for reasons of morality, hobble research on the still distressingly long catalogue of human ills. What, one may ask, is the morality of such a dog-in-the-manger attitude?

Accepting the thesis that continued animal research is essential, it can also be agreed that there must be standards and principles to ensure the proper use and welfare of the animals. There are. The minimal level of assurance is with the self-interest of investigators, who understand that the validity of their research may be compromised by the use of animals that are not healthy or have not had proper care. In fact, the vast majority of scientists also have compassion and humane concerns for the animals they use daily in their work. Now, in addition to these self-imposed standards, there are laws and regulations that require the humane treatment of animals used in research. These standards are embraced by funding agencies, research institutions, private and industrial organizations, and individual scientists. When the National Institute of Health was established in 1930, there was in the Office of the Director an "Inspector for Humane Treatment of Animals." Today, institutional facilities and research programs are operated in accordance with the Public Health Service (PHS) "Guide for the Care and Use of Laboratory Animals," with the Animal Welfare Act (P.L. 89-544, as amended by P.L. 91-579 and P.L. 94-279), and with various state and local laws. The PHS assurance system for guaranteeing adherence to standards for animal facilities, for the care and treatment of animals, and for their appropriateness for a given research protocol has been remarkably successful and demonstrates that scientists and the institutions in which they work have both the capacity and the willingness to act responsibly.

COMMERCIAL, ECONOMIC, AND SOCIAL IMPERATIVES

The nation's biomedical research enterprise not only has brought about profound improvements in human health but also has developed new medical technologies and procedures that have become integrated into the health care system. The instrumentation required for these new technologies has led to industrial incentives for their manufacture and to cognate medical incentives for their use. Indeed, the rapid development of instrumentation has outrun considerations of cost-effectiveness, diagnostic need, safety, and efficacy. Technology assessment has developed as a distinct discipline (with its own need for research) but has not yet reached a significant level of effectiveness. The consequences of technological development derived from biomedical research thus raise another set of economic, social, and ethical questions.

Approximately $600 billion was spent in the United States in 1990 for health care services. This amounts to about 12 percent of the gross national product (GNP), and this figure is continuing to climb in an almost uncontrolled fashion. Although the U.S. health care system has been called the best in the world, there is increasing anxiety that its mounting costs will erode national prosperity, and there are other, more specific, concerns. Most Americans receive health insurance through their jobs, and many others are covered by the government, through Medicaid or Medicare, which now pays 40 percent of the nation's health bills. Nevertheless, 33 million Americans, or one in eight, have no health insurance.

The soaring cost of health care—and consequent increasing insurance rates—has in part been ascribed to the introduction of more and more technologies in a system that has few internal controls and is quite content to let the government or the insurance carriers pay the bill. Many organizations, state and local governments, insurance companies, and the federal government are addressing the overall problem, and various plans have been put forth, all with the avowed aim of assuring access to health care for all of our citizens while controlling costs. The president's budget for 1992 includes a proposal to cut some $20 billion from projected Medicare fees to hospitals and doctors over the next five years. The Office of Management and Budget (OMB) is also considering the establishment of a computerized system to collect and maintain information on which Americans have private or employer-based health insurance. This system would be used to ensure that private insurance, when required by law, pays medical bills before Medicaid and other government programs are charged. Under this proposal, employers would be required to show, on Internal Revenue Service W-2 forms, which employees are covered by insurance.

Biomedical research has contributed to this national economic problem by constantly developing new medical technologies—new techniques, drugs, equipment, procedures—that are quickly taken up by those who provide medical care. As a consequence, a technology industry of considerable size has grown up, which has created new relationships between the research and health service communities, on the one hand, and the commercial sector, on the other. The industrial sector manufactures and markets the new products to an eager health service sector that is ever-anxious to have the latest and the best in health care gadgetry. Despite its economic consequences, the flow of new technology cannot, in good conscience, be halted or seriously impeded, for that would deprive the public of the new and beneficial procedures that the biomedical research enterprise was intended to develop. The problem can and should, however, be mitigated by requiring researchers and health care providers to assess the appropriateness and effectiveness of the use of these procedures and to set forth national policies and standards for their use. A useful step in this direction is the 1985 report of the Institute of Medicine (IOM), "Assessing Medical Technologies" (Institute of Medicine, Committee for Evaluating Medical Technologies 1985).

The emergence of *medical imaging,* a technology that has evolved to the point of yielding unprecedented information without the necessity of invasive techniques, is a prime example of the cost-benefit problem. The CAT scanner was developed in the early 1970s, as the result of research in many diverse fields. It represented a great advance over the old x-ray machine but cost $500 per scan in the early days. The cost of the scanner itself was initially about $300,000 but is now over a million dollars. The CAT scanner quickly spread to industrialized nations. In the United States there are over 2000 scanners, representing a capital investment of more than a billion dollars and operating expenses of a like amount. As valuable as this instrument is, it is not yet definitely known what kinds of patients justify the expense of the scan. The aforementioned IOM study indicated that millions of CAT head scans were performed each year for people with uncomplicated headaches.

MRI emerged in the early 1970s and allows the visualization of both hard and soft tissues. It is cheaper and safer than exploratory surgery, which might have been required to determine the need for and extent of further surgery. These machines cost millions of dollars and have a hefty annual operating cost. A typical imaging visit costs patients from $600 to $1000. As with the CAT scan, many experts in technology assessment claim that the procedure is often overused, often producing information that is of marginal value. MRI is, in fact, the center of a national debate over costs and ethics, as reported by Robert Pear in a 1991 article in the *New York Times*. Pear reported that the city of Atlanta had one MRI machine in 1984. The city now has at least thirty, and most are owned by doctors, more often than not the same doctors who send their patients for scans. Critics maintain that this practice is a clear conflict of interest and that it promotes an overuse of procedures. Defenders of the practice claim that the service enhances the quality of medical care and makes the new technology more widely available. An important consideration is that the practice protects the physician from malpractice claims by a public demanding "perfect" medical care. Similar opportunities for entrepreneurism in the practice of medicine are increasing, and, as is shown later in this chapter, a similar trend is emerging for the bench scientist.

Despite the spiraling costs of medical care and the development of new technologies that are sometimes used indiscriminately and for personal gain, a more serious economic problem arises from the fact that people are living longer. The population of aged people has increased at a phenomenal rate (Proceedings of the Regional Institutes on Geriatrics and Medical Education 1983). Since about 1950, the population of those sixty-five and older has grown twice as fast as the population as a whole, and it is projected that this cohort will comprise 18 percent of the total population by 2035. The number of individuals eighty-five and over is the fastest-growing segment within the aged population. Demographers (Elmer-Dewitt 1990) predict, however, that this increase in life expectancy is coming to an end and that the disorderly deterioration that comes with aging will stabilize, resulting in an average life expectancy of eighty-five years. This prediction may, however, have to be revised if the genes that cause cells to wear out are discovered, understood, and subject to manipulation.

As described in the 1989 Report of the U.S. Department of Health and Human Services Advisory Panel on Alzheimer's disease, the dementing disorders of the increasing aged population demonstrate in a dramatic way the social, economic, and ethical dilemmas that result from the successes of biomedical research. For many in the aging population, these disorders gradually lead to the loss of mental and functional abilities. Affected individuals have memory loss and other intellectual impairments that leave them confused, disoriented, and incapable of communicating normally. In time, they become dependent on others for their personal needs and safety. The report goes on to say that "the personal tragedy of Alzheimer's disease and other dementias is that they dissolve the mind and steal the humanity of the victim, leaving a body from which the person has largely been removed."

Alzheimer's disease, the most prevalent of the dementing disorders, is estimated to account for 4 million cases annually, at a cost of over $40 billion for the care of these patients. These costs can be expected to escalate as longevity continues to increase. Is it right, is it moral for science to prolong life with its accompanying relentless reduction in function and gradual disintegration? As with other diseases that accompany the aging process, biomedical research offers the only hope for their alleviation, cure, and prevention.

The reality of life is a succession of generations, each in subjection to the place and time of its existence. In this century, among those born before drugs were developed to treat hypertension, or before the polio vaccine or open heart surgery, many were destined for early death or permanent affliction. Even they were better off than those who lived before the advent of anesthesia and aseptic surgery, all of whom had to endure the pain of the knife without the benefit of these advances. Further, these differences are not a matter of time alone; the matter of place, both geographic and on the social ladder, also determines what sort of health care and medical treatment will be available. There are still many who live under primitive conditions in remote or so-called underdeveloped areas; there also are many, to our shame, who live in poverty and neglect under our very noses. Biomedical research can only offer the possibilities of treatments, cures, and preventions; it is the responsibility of society at large to ensure that future generations will be benefited by them in a more uniform and equitable manner than is true today. That, too, is an important moral imperative.

SCIENCE FOR SALE?

The phrase "Science for Sale" is not original, but it aptly brings us to the underlying thesis of the chapters to follow. During a visit to the National Institutes of Health in 1983, the Secretary of the Department of Health and Human Services declared that "NIH is an island of objective and pristine research excellence, untainted by commercialization influences. . . . I will do all that I can to make it attractive to work here for the star scientists." By 1991, the NIH had established an Office of Technology Transfer, had developed 140 cooperative research and development agreements (CRADAs) with industry, had received about $3 million in royalties, and had relaxed its policies to permit NIH scientists to engage in compensated consulting for industrial organizations.

This dramatic change in the intramural programs of the world's premier research institution mirrored similar but more extensive changes in the academic community. Both are due to the accelerating alliances between biomedical research and industry, sparked by the revolutionary advances in molecular biology and the growing field of biotechnology. There are many variations of growing university-industry relationships (Office of Technology Assessment Task Force Report 1990). The simplest form encompasses faculty consulting and research relationships, which can range from informal collaborations to formal consulting and research support with patent and licensing agreements. The university itself may have its own relationships with corporations. These may involve long-term contracts (such as the long-standing agreement between Monsanto and Washington University in St. Louis), university-controlled research parks, and many other variations. By 1991, more than 100 American universities had started financing new companies to exploit the research findings of their faculties for commercial advantage. Individual faculty members and universities can make money, potentially big money, from science.

We are probably just at the tip of the iceberg of commercial opportunity in biomedical research. Recombinant-DNA technology has already led to the production of human insulin, human growth hormone, interferon, antihemophilic factors, vaccines, monoclonal antibodies, erythropoietin, tissue plasminogen activator (TPA), and many other substances. The biotechnology industry is flourishing today as no other segment in the health care industry. Biotechnology sales reached $5.8 billion in 1991 and are projected to reach $50 billion by the year 2000. The Human Genome Project offers incredible possibilities for alleviating or controlling disease through human gene therapy or the use of gene products. It can be predicted that these changes will, in time, change the practice of medicine with profound changes on the quality of life for people everywhere.

Just in the past five decades, biomedical research has moved from a time when most basic science researchers performed what many call "disinterested" research, research pursued for the sake of knowledge acquisition, to the present era of megaprojects and widespread interest in the commercialization of academic research. There have always been modest interactions with industry, particularly in the area of drug development, but nothing approaching the present and growing state of university-industry relationships. This transition has been accompanied by other important changes in the public and scientific sectors. The public governance of science has been on the ascendancy, such that science is continually under scrutiny by the press, the public, and the lawmakers. There is increased competition for available federal dollars for new investigators, increased costs for research, and a general need to renew the research infrastructure. All this is occurring amid unprecedented scientific opportunities. In this changing culture of university research, there is a rising tide of university-industry relationships. These relationships have accelerated technology transfer but have had profound impact on the functions and structure of universities, provoking a new set of moral, ethical, and legal concerns.

The changes in faculty behavior associated with industrial collaboration are an area of intense public concern. Questions have been raised about such matters as secrecy and reduction in intellectual exchange, shifts in research toward areas of interest to industry, delay in publication of findings that may have commercial applications, use of graduate students in the pursuit of research being pursued for industry, and other reductions in the commitment and responsibility for teaching and service. An early study by Blumenthal et al. (1986) suggested that these risks had been, for the most part, contained, at least for the period of the study. Universities will have to be increasingly vigilant as they continue to target their efforts toward economic development and technological innovation.

A major national debate has centered around whether investigators should have equity in any company for which they are engaged in research. The debate has been fueled by headline cases of conflicts of interest. Fortunately, the U.S. Public Health Services has had a policy on conflict of interest in place for many years. That policy requires institutions receiving federal funds for research to establish safeguards to prevent employees, consultants, or members of governing bodies from using their positions for private financial gain for themselves, for family members, or for others with whom they have business ties. This policy also requires each institution to have written policy guidelines on conflicts of interest and their avoidance. We examine here their application and utility, for it is only through the promulgation of clearly enunciated, publicized, and enforced policies that the transfer of knowledge can take place for the public good.

A discussion of *moral imperatives*—a term that has here been rather loosely used as a synonym for "necessity"—must accept the premise that morality is not an absolute but a relative concept. Actions and views that conform to the accepted standards of right and wrong are considered moral, but what is accepted will, of course, depend on when, where, and under what circumstances the judgment on morality is made. There are obvious examples: Fifty years ago, premarital cohabitation was socially unacceptable, yet now it is more the norm than the exception; in Arab countries, a veil must cover a woman's face in public, whereas in the West, a bikini covers almost nothing; in peacetime, killing is a crime, but in war, it is a patriotic duty. Moreover, as a moral judgment is a mix of what is considered right or good and what is considered wrong or evil, the acceptable proportion of good to evil will fluctuate in accordance with how strongly the good is desired. There has always been controversy about what is moral and what is not: "I find the doctors and the sages Have differ'd in all climes and ages, And two in fifty scarce agree On what is pure morality" (Thomas Moore, 1779–1852).

Strictly speaking, morality must also be the product of consensus because it purports to be a standard conforming to the mores, customs, and conventions of the community. An individual can be more ethical or more righteous than another but cannot be a bit more or a bit less moral. The current debates about abortion, contraception, animal rights, gene therapy, and so forth, seen in this light, are not about morality, for there is no clear societal consensus on their rightness or wrongness, their good or evil. The debates are about policy in the face of conflicting ethical judgments, religious beliefs, and prejudices.

The moral imperative of biomedical research is a function not of its specific components but of the importance and desirability—on which there is a very broad consensus—of reaping the benefits of the requisite knowledge and more effective techniques for preventing and curing disease that are, at long last, rapidly becoming available. This prospect, to misquote Shakespeare slightly, "shines like a good deed in a naughty world."

The exciting prospects for preventive and therapeutic medicine are the more welcome and, perhaps, the more urgent because they come at a time when the human race has little other ground for confidence or cheer. The editors of *Time* devoted the cover story of the June 10, 1991, edition to a dismal catalog of the "evil" that now exists in the world: environmental, social, economic and political, of which, unfortunately, the environmental may be the least remediable and the most threatening.

A century ago, irresponsible concern for profits over prudence began to have cumulative consequences that are now beginning to pose a threat to the survival of life on this planet. The manufacture of carcinogenic chemicals, ill-protected hazardous waste, acid rain, air pollution, holes in the ozone layer, pollution of ground and surface waters, ocean-floor pollution, oil spills on beaches, and the destruction of the rain forests are all taking their toll on the environment and having direct and indirect effects on human health.

On the domestic front, we have, historically, also had laws, policies, and institutions that favored the protection of property over the welfare of people. Treatment of the two has often been inequitable. What was sauce for the goose was not always sauce for the gander, or, as one early critic of real estate development put it,

> The law deals hard with man or woman
> Who steals a goose from off the common
> But lets the greater villain loose
> Who steals the common from the goose.

There were fire departments before there were health departments. There is federal deposit insurance for the money people have in the banks but no health insurance for 30 million Americans. As-yet-uncounted billions will be spent to repair the mismanagement of financial institutions and to improve the safety of wealth; in comparison, only a pittance is available for repairing the misfortunes of ordinary people and for improving their quality of life—welfare, sheltering the homeless, education, health care, and, yes, medical research.

There is now the prospect—actually already under way—that big-science biomedical research will follow in the footsteps of the military, the nuclear, and the space establishments to become part of a medical industrial complex in which the researchers, the health care providers, and the manufacturers who supply them will be closely linked. There is merit in such an arrangement, in possible economies of scale, in more effective communication about problems that arise in a segment of the triumvirate, in speeding up the transfer of technology, and in the easier accessibility of facilities and resources. However, there are also obvious dangers: that the larger enterprise will become more bureaucratic, that decision making may lie in the wrong hands, that a more businesslike atmosphere will prevail that is inimical to intellectual pursuits, and, especially, that efforts will be directed to areas where the biggest or quickest profits may be expected. Medical schools, universities, hospitals, clinics, and independent research facilities—not to mention their faculties and staffs—all have financial problems that, in the immediate future, are likely to get worse. The temptation to turn hard-pressed nonprofit institutions into money-making enterprises will be very great and hard to resist.

On the other hand, a well-run cooperative venture between the research, the service, and the industrial sectors that does not lose sight of the fundamental purposes of each component might set a pattern for joint approaches to some of the other major problems that need to be solved. The present state of play, its potential, its weaknesses, and its probable future direction are discussed in this volume.

To those who devote their lives to the search for more effective ways of countering disease and disability and to those who diligently use that knowledge to care for the sick and disabled, we owe our grateful thanks and best wishes.

Cura ut valeas!

REFERENCES

Bible. Genesis 1:28, King James Version.
Bloch, H. 1987. Man's curiosity about food digestion: An historical overview. *Journal of the National Medical Association.* 79(110): 1123–226.
Blumenthal, D. et al. 1986. University-industry research relationships in biotechnology: Implications for the university. *Science.* 232: 1361–66.
Breo, D. L. 1990. MD's of the millennium: The dozen who made a difference. *Journal of the American Medical Association.* 263(1): 108–13.
Covey, H. C. 1989. Old age portrayed by the ages-of-life models from the Middle Ages to the 16th century. *Gerontologist.* 29(5): 692–97.
Dekker, T. 1968. Marcus B. Strauss: *Familiar Medical Quotations.* pp. 202, 203, 498.
Descartes, R. 1968. Marcus B. Strauss: *Familiar Medical Quotations.* pp. 202, 203, 498.
Elmer-Dewitt, P. 1990. You should live so long. *Time.* November 12, p. 86.
Encyclopedia Britannica, 14th ed. 1929. Vol. 11, p. 585.
Encyclopedia Britannica, 15th ed. 1974. Vol. 2, p. 827.
Henderson, L. J. 1964. Quoted in *New England Journal of Medicine.* 270: 449.
Institute of Medicine, Committee for Evaluating Medical Technologies in Clinical Use. 1985. *Assessing Medical Technologies.* Washington, D.C.: National Academy of Sciences Press.
Major, R. H. 1954. *A History of Medicine,* Vol. 1. Springfield, Illinois: Charles C Thomas.

de Montaigne, M. 1968. Marcus B. Strauss: *Familiar Medical Quotations.* pp. 202, 203, 498.

Office of Technology Assessment Task Force Report. 1990. *New Developments in Biotechnology: Ownership of Human Tissues and Cells.* Philadelphia: J. P. Lippincott.

Panati, C. 1989. *Panati's Extraordinary Endings of Practically Everything and Everybody.* New York: Harper & Row.

Pear, R. 1991. When healers are entrepreneurs: A debate over costs and ethics. *New York Times.* June 2, p. 1.

Proceedings of the Regional Institutes on Geriatrics and Medical Education. 1983. Washington, D.C.: Association of American Medical Colleges.

Report of the U.S. Department of Health and Human Services Advisory Panel on Alzheimer's Disease. 1989. DHHS Publication No. (ADM) 89-1644. Washington, D.C.: U.S. Government Printing Office.

U.S. Department of Health and Human Services. 1992. *1992 Monthly Vital Statistics Report,* 40: Suppl. 2 No 8

Vischer, M. B. 1975. *Ethical Constraints and Imperatives in Medical Research.* Springfield, Illinois: Charles C Thomas.

Wattenberg, B. J., and the United States Bureau of the Census. 1970. *The Statistical History of the United States: From Colonial Times to the Present.* New York: Basic Books.

Woodward, T. 1989. Religion and medicine. *Maryland Medical Journal* 38(7): 568–72.

2 • The Funding of Basic and Clinical Biomedical Research

Alicia K. Dustira

Funding is never far from the thoughts of any research scientist. The size and source of research funding can affect every aspect of the research process—its scope, its pace, its quality, and even its direction. Indeed, in many ways, research funding forms the underpinnings of biomedical science, always necessary, often unseen, and never without some effect on how scientific knowledge is acquired. To understand the state of biomedical research in this country, therefore, we must understand how research is funded and how that support has changed over the past fifty years.

Since World War II, the funding of biomedical research in the United States has changed enormously. Before the war, government funding represented less than 10 percent of all money for biomedical research, with most financial resources coming from industry and philanthropic organizations. After the war, government funding steadily increased until federal monies composed more than half of all biomedical research funds.

Now, however, we are witnessing a reversal of this trend. In the past decade, there have been sharp and significant changes in the direction of both industry and government funding. Industry support grew from 29 to 46 percent of the total national investment in health research and development between 1979 and 1990. In contrast, the federal government's portion of the nation's support for biomedical research fell from 60 to 44 percent during that time.

A variety of factors explains this shift. Large federal deficits in the 1980s put tremendous pressures on all parts of the federal budget, including research. The passage of the Gramm-Rudman-Hollings Deficit

Reduction Act in 1985 further intensified the pressures for all the federal agencies to remain within specific fiscal guidelines. Also, the appearance of exciting new applications for the results of biomedical research, including biotechnology, fostered increased industrial investment in biomedical research. This chapter briefly documents the history of the changing support for biomedical research and summarizes the current state of support provided by federal, state, and local governments, by industry, and by private, nonprofit organizations.

THE HISTORY OF CHANGING SUPPORT
FOR BIOMEDICAL RESEARCH

The concept that scholarship and advanced research training should be conducted jointly in institutions of higher learning has been a major tenet of most U.S. universities and medical centers for more than a century. This dual emphasis on new knowledge and pedagogy has established a unique interdependence between education and research in this country. Institutions of higher learning educate new generations of teachers, physicians, investigators, and other professionals, while producing fundamental knowledge for the advancement of science and for social, economic, and cultural development.

Before World War II, academic research was sponsored primarily by philanthropic foundations and industries. For the most part, foundations awarded block grants to major private universities, while industries generally underwrote programmatic grants in their areas of commercial interest (Government-University-Industry Research Roundtable 1989).

In 1940, industry contributed over half of the estimated $45 million spent on biomedical research in the United States. More than one third came from philanthropy, either through earnings on endowments or grants from foundations. The federal government's investment that year was less than 7 percent of the total ($3 million), and was spent mostly in its own laboratories (Bloom and Randolph 1990, Ginzberg and Dutka 1989) (Figure 2.1).

World War II changed the country's attitudes toward government support of research. It was clear that a key role during the war was played by scientists, including medical scientists who reduced battle casualties and protected our troops from infectious diseases (Ginzberg and Dutka 1989). This experience illustrated the important contributions that scientific research could make and led to the postwar expansion of federal investment in research, particularly basic research. This

Figure 2.1. Sources of funding for biomedical research and development (R&D) (in millions of dollars).

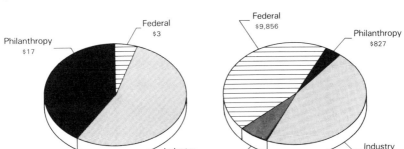

1940
total: $45 million

1990
total: $22.5 billion

Source: Data from U.S. Department of Health and Human Services (DHHS), Public Health Service (PHS) 1990.

expansion fostered the creation of the system whereby grants and contracts are awarded to institutions based on scientific merit (Bloom and Randolph 1990, Ginzberg and Dutka 1989), and federal funding for health research grew dramatically.

Currently, federal programs account for 44 percent of the total national expenditures for health research and development in the United States (U.S. Department of Health and Human Services [DHHS], Public Health Service [PHS] 1990) (Figure 2.2). Of the more than $60 billion that the federal government spent on general scientific research and development in 1989, nearly $9 billion supported biomedical research and development (Bloom and Randolph 1990). Nearly three quarters of the federal government's support for biomedical research comes through programs of the National Institutes of Health (NIH) in the U.S. DHHS. The other federal departments and agencies that have noteworthy budgets for health sciences research include the Alcohol, Drug Abuse, and Mental Health Administration (ADAMHA) in DHHS, the National Science Foundation (NSF), and the Departments of Defense, Energy, and Veterans Affairs (DOD, DOE, and DVA, respectively) (Bloom and Randolph 1990) (Figure 2.3).

Two thirds of federally sponsored biomedical research in the United States is conducted in colleges and universities, medical

Figure 2.2. Funding for biomedical R&D, by source, 1980–90 (in millions of dollars). Constant dollars (fiscal year = 1980) are calculated using the biomedical R&D price index.

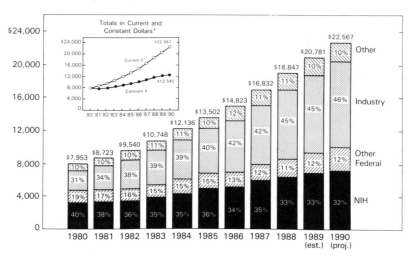

Source: Data from U.S. DHHS, PHS 1990.

schools, and research organizations. Approximately one quarter is performed in federal laboratories (Figure 2.4). In contrast, more than three quarters of all industrially sponsored biomedical research and development is performed within corporate facilities (U.S. DHHS, PHS 1990).

Figure 2.3. Federal funding for biomedical R&D, 1989 (in millions of dollars).

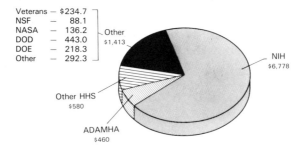

Source: Data from U.S. DHHS, PHS 1990; Bloom and Randolph 1990.

Figure 2.4. The distribution of federal funding for biomedical R&D, 1989 (in millions of dollars).

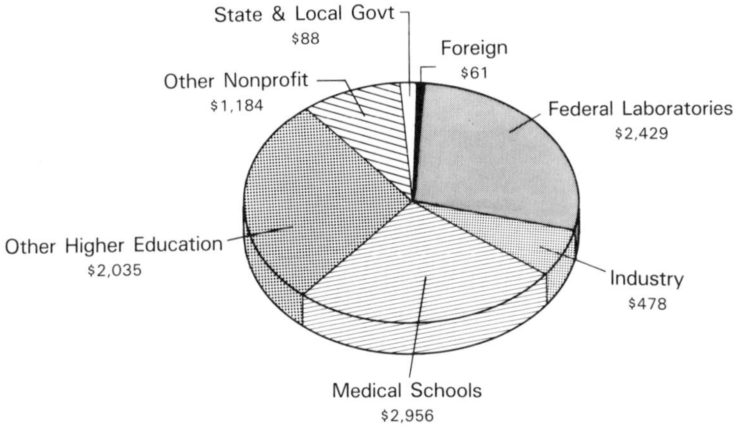

State & Local Govt
$88

Foreign
$61

Other Nonprofit
$1,184

Federal Laboratories
$2,429

Other Higher Education
$2,035

Industry
$478

Medical Schools
$2,956

Source: Data from U.S. DHHS, PHS 1990.

NIH SUPPORT FOR BIOMEDICAL RESEARCH

Before World War II, nearly all federally funded biomedical research was carried out in government laboratories. In the two decades following the war, Congress not only significantly increased funding for health research, but it also changed the way that most of the scientific research in the United States was conducted and organized. The NIH, a part of PHS, began supporting research through ever-increasing extramural grant and fellowship programs. In addition, major expansion of U.S. biomedical research facilities during the late 1950s to 1970s was made possible through a new NIH construction authority (Bloom and Randolph 1990).

The U.S. Congress dramatically increased funding for biomedical research between 1945 and 1965, a period during which appropriations for NIH rose from $26 million to $4 billion in constant 1988 dollars (Figure 2.5). Although the rate of growth in funding for health research slowed after 1965, NIH continued to expand its role in research during the 1960s and 1970s (Bloom and Randolph 1990).

Inflationary pressures in the 1970s slowed the real growth of the NIH budget (Figure 2.5). During the 1980s, NIH appropriations increased an average of 10 percent per year, resulting in a 2 percent per

Figure 2.5. NIH appropriations, 1945–91 (in current and constant 1988 dollars).

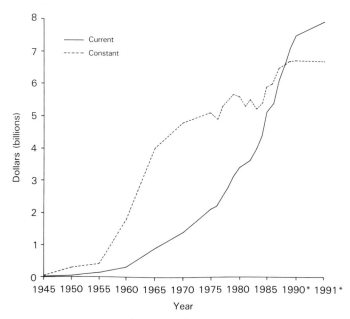

Source: Data from Bloom and Randolph 1990.
Note: Constant 1988 dollars are calculated using the biomedical R&D price index.
(*indicates estimates.)

year growth in constant dollars between 1981 and 1989 (Bloom and Randolph 1990) (Figure 2.6).

NIH currently consists of thirteen institutes, two support divisions, the Clinical Center, the Fogarty International Center, four specialized centers, and the National Library of Medicine. Unlike many other federal agencies, nearly 80 percent of the NIH budget supports research and training outside of the government, usually at universities or medical schools. These funds are primarily awarded through competitive peer-review processes. Of the remaining 20 percent of the NIH budget, most is spent for intramural activities of the thirteen institutes. The intramural programs support basic and clinical research, scientist training, and application of research findings to improve medical care (Bloom and Randolph 1990).

Investigator-initiated research and development (R&D) grants are considered a key feature of NIH research support, and this portion of the NIH portfolio is watched very closely by the extramural commu-

Figure 2.6. NIH appropriations, 1981–91 (in current and constant 1988 dollars).

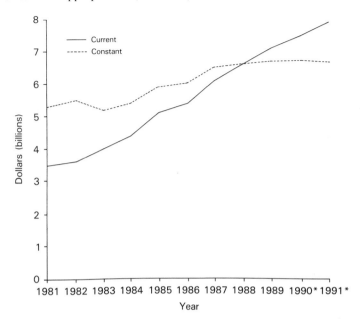

Source: Data from Bloom and Randolph 1990.
Note: Constant 1988 dollars are calculated using the biomedical R&D price index.
(*indicates estimates.)

nity. In particular, those grants awarded to individual investigators (R01s), are often the focus of much analysis and heated debate regarding the appropriate level of support for individual scientists in any given year.

During the 1970s, the commitments to ongoing projects increased, partly due to an NIH policy of gradually increasing the average *award period*. Increasing the length of a grant was intended to increase the stability of research support, and it was hoped that it would reduce the number of multiple applications submitted to NIH. In theory, longer grant periods also would reduce the amount of time an investigator spent writing new proposals and would relieve some of the administrative burdens on NIH in processing and reviewing applications.

At the same time, however, research costs continued to escalate, and the growth in the numbers of new and competing proposals submitted to NIH each year continued unabated. Because the total NIH budget did not increase sufficiently to compensate for these trends, this tended to reduce the number of new and competing grants that could be awarded in any given year.

In addition, there were noticeable yearly fluctuations in the number of new proposals funded during the 1970s, caused by variations in commitments to ongoing grants. These fluctuations engendered grave concern within NIH and in the extramural community, and they led the U.S. Congress and the Administration to agree on a policy that specified the minimum number of new and competing NIH and ADAMHA grants to be funded each year—known as the "stabilization policy."

The stabilization policy was in effect from 1981 to 1988. Despite increased appropriations from Congress, the funds available were never sufficient to fully fund the specified numbers of new grants. In order to meet the target numbers, NIH and ADAMHA had to resort to across-the-board cuts in funding ongoing research projects as well as new awards. In addition, NIH shifted more of its extramural portfolio to supporting R&D grants during the 1980s, mostly at the expense of extramural contracts and training (Figure 2.7).

Although the policy of specifying the minimum number of new and competing grants to be awarded per year was dropped from appropri-

Figure 2.7. The allocation of NIH extramural awards, 1972–88 (in millions of dollars).

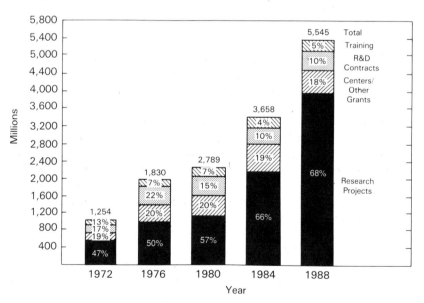

Source: Data from Bloom and Randolph 1990.

ations language for fiscal years (FYs) 1989 and 1990, anxiety about this segment of the NIH budget continued. Testimony and letter-writing campaigns heralding a crisis in biomedical research funding caused the U.S. Congressional appropriations committee to express their concern over the lack of a clear plan for cost management and control, as well as a concern for stability and predictability of funding. When Congress gave NIH nearly $1 billion more for FY 1991 than the Administration requested, it also directed NIH to respond to a ten-point plan to redistribute and control research costs. Congress expected to see this plan as part of the 1992 budget request, as well as appropriate modifications that are compatible with the goals of predictability and stability.

BIOMEDICAL RESEARCH SUPPORT FROM OTHER FEDERAL AGENCIES

Alcohol, Drug Abuse, and Mental Health Administration (ADAMHA)

In 1973, the National Institute of Alcohol Abuse and Alcoholism (NIAAA) and the National Institute on Drug Abuse (NIDA) were merged with the National Institute of Mental Health (NIMH) to form ADAMHA. In this way, ADAMHA became a comparable agency to NIH within the PHS, with a total budget similar to some of the larger NIH institutes ($1.56 billion in FY 1989).

In addition to conducting and supporting biomedical research and training, ADAMHA funds demonstration projects, clinical training, and treatment, prevention, and public information activities. ADAMHA's programs for research and training, as well as its peer-review process, are nearly identical to those at NIH.

Throughout the 1970s, ADAMHA's budget grew in parallel with the NIH budget. In the early 1980s, however, cuts in social sciences research and community programs caused the total ADAMHA appropriations to shrink during that time. Community programs still account for more than 50 percent of the ADAMHA budget. From 1977 until 1989, the research component of the ADAMHA portfolio grew from less than 20 to 35 percent of the total (Bloom and Randolph 1990) (Figure 2.8).

Centers for Disease Control (CDC)

The Centers for Disease Control are charged with (a) assisting state and local health officials and other organizations to reduce the spread of communicable diseases, (b) protecting the public from diseases or health conditions that can be minimized, (c) providing protec-

Figure 2.8. ADAMHA budget allocations, 1977–89 (in millions of dollars).

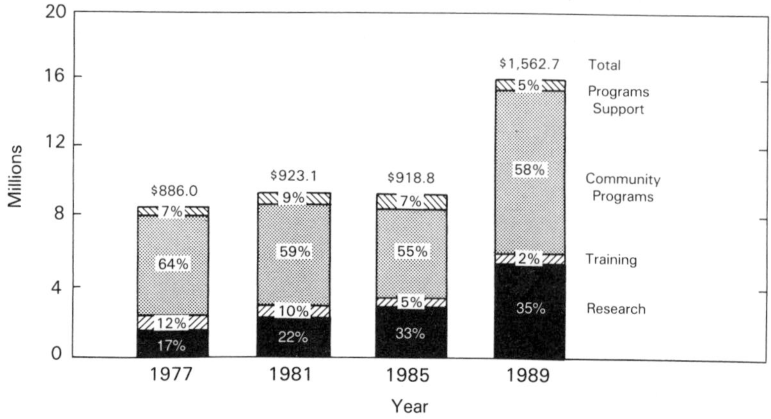

Source: Data from Bloom and Randolph 1990.

tion from particular environmental hazards, and (d) improving occupational health and safety. About 90 percent of the total CDC budget is spent for nonresearch activities, mostly through block grants to states. In FY 1989, $100.6 million was spent on CDC biomedical research (Bloom and Randolph 1990).

Department of Veterans Affairs (DVA)

The Department of Veterans Affairs provides health care to veterans through its hospitals and centers throughout the country, and it has developed research programs related to that mission. The DVA research budget supports medical research (85 percent), rehabilitation research (11 percent), and health services R&D (4 percent). All R&D projects are peer reviewed. In FY 1989, $207.5 million was appropriated for the DVA research budget. Career development activities are part of the research budget as well, including some salary support for training young physician investigators (Bloom and Randolph 1990).

National Science Foundation (NSF)

The National Science Foundation was created in 1950 as an independent government agency to promote scientific progress through basic research in all fields of science and engineering. Approximately 14 percent of its $2.4 billion budget is allocated to the biological, behavioral, and social sciences. Because NSF's mission excludes human disease-related research, NSF's support for biological research primarily focuses on biological processes and questions that can help build a foundation of knowledge useful to biomedical research (Bloom and Randolph 1990).

National Aeronautics and Space Administration (NASA)

The National Aeronautics and Space Administration has a small, highly specialized life sciences research program, created to support NASA's manned space programs. Although most of NASA's life sciences research funds are spent on intramural programs, it does award a limited number of $50,000 to $60,000 grants to investigators in academia (Bloom and Randolph 1990).

Department of Defense (DOD)

The Department of Defense conducts biomedical research important to national security. The Army, Navy, and Air Force all have biomedical research programs related to their mission and needs. The Army receives approximately 80 percent of the DOD funds allocated for biomedical research, spending about $250 million per year on medical research related to military disease hazards, biological warfare defense, combat casualty care, and so forth. The Office of Naval Research received $36 million in 1989 for research in the biological, medical, cognitive, and neural sciences. In the same year, the Air Force received $17.1 million to support research in neuroscience, experimental psychology, toxicology, radiation biology, and cardiovascular physiology (Bloom and Randolph 1990).

Department of Energy (DOE)

The Department of Energy sponsors research on the health effects of exposure to radiation and other hazardous substances, and it makes substantial contributions toward mapping the human genome (in cooperation with NIH). Most of the biomedical research sponsored by DOE is conducted in its national laboratories. In 1990, DOE allocated $330 million for research programs in the biological, environmental, and life sciences (Bloom and Randolph 1990).

INDUSTRY SUPPORT FOR BIOMEDICAL RESEARCH

Before World War II, industry funded more than half of all health sciences research in the United States. Following the war, industry's portion of support, while continuing to increase, was outpaced by the investment of the federal government (Bloom and Randolph 1990).

Industry is again playing an increasingly important role in health sciences research, primarily in research related to product development. Biotechnology firms and manufacturers of pharmaceuticals, medical devices, and instrumentation are examples of the types of industries engaged in health sciences R&D (Bloom and Randolph 1990).

Starting in the 1970s, widespread concern that U.S. industry was losing its competitive edge in world markets fostered changes in public policy and a substantial increase in U.S. industrial investment in R&D (Bloom and Randolph 1990). Industry's portion of the total national investment in health R&D grew from 29 percent in 1979 to 46 percent by 1990 (U.S. DHHS, PHS 1990).

It has been estimated that nearly 80 percent of industrial R&D is development, whereas basic research accounts for only 5 percent. The remaining 15 percent is categorized as applied research (Bloom and Randolph 1990). Of the total industrial expenditures on health R&D, only a small fraction (4 percent) supports research at institutions of higher education.

An NSF survey of the biotechnology industry estimated that it invested $1.4 billion on R&D in 1987, while pharmaceutical manufacturers alone spent almost $5.4 billion. Industry is the most rapidly growing portion of the national investment in biomedical R&D, and the total industrial investment has exceeded the NIH budget since 1982 (Bloom and Randolph 1990).

Although exact figures on total industrial investment in biomedical R&D are not available, there are aggregate measures available from an annual survey of the Pharmaceutical Manufacturers Association (PMA) (PMA 1990), from NSF's Survey of Biotechnology Research and Development Activities in Industry, and from a group of companies included in *Business Week's* annual "R&D Scoreboard" (Buderi, Carey, et al. 1991).

The Pharmaceutical Industry

The member firms of the PMA budgeted $7.3 billion in 1989 on R&D and expected to spend more than $8 billion in 1990. More than 80 percent of these funds are spent in the United States, with 16.4 percent of the total spent on research done outside the firm funding the research (PMA 1990). Pharmaceutical company R&D expenditures in the United States represent about 17 percent of total U.S. pharmaceutical sales, up from 11.6 percent in 1983. Ninety-seven percent of company R&D funds were spent on human-use pharmaceuticals, with the remaining 3 percent spent on products for animal use. Nearly three quarters of company R&D funds are spent on investigations related to cardiovascular products, anti-infectives, and cancer and nervous-system drugs (PMA 1990).

Eighty-three percent of pharmaceutical company R&D funds are spent for R&D of new products, with 17 percent allocated for improvement of existing products. About half of all pharmaceutical company R&D expenditures are allocated to biological screening and pharmacological testing, clinical evaluation, and synthesis and extraction. Manufacturers are devoting more than a quarter of their R&D funds to the clinical evaluation of drugs (Figure 2.9).

For the most part, the pharmaceutical industry depends on academia to provide new scientific talent. Pharmaceutical companies increased their employment of R&D personnel approximately 5 percent per year between 1984 and 1988. PMA member firms employed 41,520 R&D personnel in 1988, with 66 percent of those being classified as scientific or professional (PMA 1990).

Though industrial investment in biomedical R&D is still growing, the rate of growth appears to have been leveling off in recent years.

Figure 2.9. The distribution of U.S. R&D funding for ethical pharmaceuticals, by function.

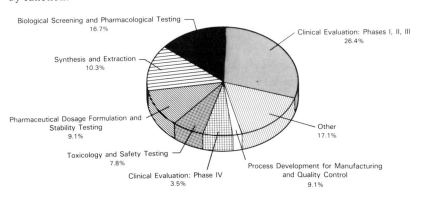

Source: Data from Pharmaceutical Manufacturers Association 1990.

This slower growth could be attributable to any number of factors, including increased international competition or mergers that compel corporations to cut costs, pressures to show short-term profits, or economic forces in a slowing economy that constrain spending on longer term investments such as R&D. Also, a reduction in tax credits for increased investment in R&D may have caused some firms to refrain from increasing their R&D expenditures. In addition, the maturation of the biotechnology industry itself may account for some of the slowed growth (Bloom and Randolph 1990).

The Biotechnology Industry

Biotechnology is one type of biomedical R&D that has received a great deal of attention in recent years. *Biotechnology* is generally defined as "any technique that uses living organisms (or parts of organisms) to make or modify products, to improve plants or animals, or to develop micro-organisms for specified uses" (Office of Technology Assessment [OTA] 1984).

Biotechnology is an ancient practice that includes such familiar applications as the use of bacterial, fungal, or yeast cultures in making cheese. However, what is commonly referred to as "biotechnology" these days means the use of recombinant-DNA techniques, cell fusion, novel bioprocessing techniques, and gene therapy to improve health or to make or modify products (Office of Management and Budget [OMB] 1991, OTA 1988). It should be noted that a significant portion, but certainly not all, of biotechnology research is biomedical in nature.

Currently, twelve federal agencies spend more than $3 billion annually for biotechnology R&D. According to OTA, the federal government was the source of nearly 60 percent of the total U.S. investment in biotechnology in 1987, with industry contributing 38 percent and states contributing approximately 2 percent. Most of the support for basic biomedical research essential to the advancement of biotechnology has come from the NIH (OMB 1991). NIH reported that nearly 22 percent, or $1.02 billion of its 1988 R&D budget, was allocated to research on developing biotechnology techniques or employing biotechnology (Bloom and Randolph 1990).

OTA carried out two surveys of biotechnology firms in 1987. In one survey of 296 biotechnology firms, 21 percent were conducting R&D in human therapeutics and 18 percent in diagnostics. In the second survey of 53 large diversified companies, 20 were involved in R&D work in diagnostics and human therapeutics. Based on these two surveys, OTA estimated that more than 70 major corporations and 403 biotechnology firms were investing in biotechnology in 1988 (Bloom and Randolph 1990). U.S. industry is spending a combined estimate of $1.5 to $2.0 billion annually in biotechnology R&D (OTA 1988).

In 1986 and 1987, corporations surveyed by NSF expected to spend at least $1 million annually on biotechnology R&D (National Science Foundation 1987). The 54 firms that responded to both surveys increased their R&D investments in biotechnology 16 percent in 1986 and 12 percent in 1987. The NSF estimated that industry invested $1.4 billion in biotechnology R&D in 1987 (Bloom and Randolph 1990).

Other Industry Surveys

Business Week has been tracking industrial R&D expenditures in an annual survey of U.S. corporations since 1976, which has included information from thirty-eight health care companies. While the survey indicated that there was a significant slowdown in the growth of R&D spending for most industries in 1990, health care reported an impressive 20 percent increase in R&D outlays, after gaining 13 percent the year before. In addition, the ratio of R&D investment to sales for the health care companies was more than 5 percent greater than the ratio cited for industry as a whole (Buderi et al. 1991).

LEGISLATION AFFECTING CORPORATE R&D

In recent years, the federal government has tried to encourage industry to increase its investment in R&D, to foster technology transfer, and to expand associations of industries with universities and government laboratories in a variety of ways (Bloom and Randolph 1990).

The 1980 Patent and Trademarks Act allowed, for the first time, universities to own patents resulting from federally sponsored research (Government-University-Industry Research Roundtable 1986). In the same year, the Stevenson-Wydler Technology Innovation Act directed all agencies with research budgets to allocate 0.5 percent of their R&D funds to industry or academia for technology transfer (Bloom and Randolph 1990).

The 1982 Small Business Innovation Development Act created a program for granting federal research funds to for-profit businesses. Currently, all federal agencies with research budgets of greater than $100 million must award 1.25 percent of their R&D funds through this program (Bloom and Randolph 1990).

The Federal Technology Transfer Act of 1986 was designed to provide incentives for collaborations between industry and federal agencies. This legislation promotes technology transfer by authorizing government laboratories to enter into cooperative research and economic development agreements (CRADAs) with other federal agencies, with state and local governments, and with both profit and nonprofit organizations (Bloom and Randolph 1990). Between 1987 and 1990, scientists at the NIH have entered into more than 200 CRADAs with private industry. Other federal agencies, such as the CDC, the Food and Drug Administration (FDA), and ADAMHA, expect to enter into CRADAs in 1991. As a result of these cooperative agreements, the number of patents filed by NIH has jumped from 90 in 1987 to more than 200 in 1989 (OMB 1990).

To foster additional investment and to stimulate technology transfer, the 1981 Economic Recovery Tax Act provided a 20 percent tax credit for incremental increases in R&D spending. With some modifications, it has been extended through the present (Bloom and Randolph 1990). The Bush Administration's FY 1992 budget included a proposal to make the 20 percent research and experimentation tax credit permanent, allowing 100 percent of research expenses to be used for computation after December 31, 1990. The 20 percent research and experimentation credit was enacted in 1989 and renewed in 1990. The budget predicts that rate to increase corporate R&D spending by about 4 percent in the 1990s. The President's budget also requests extension of tax rules that govern allocation of foreign and domestic R&D expenditures for companies with foreign operations. The Administration's proposal would allow 100 percent of U.S. expenditures to be covered, rather than the current 75 percent (OMB 1991).

THE DEVELOPMENT OF INTERACTIONS
BETWEEN INDUSTRY AND UNIVERSITIES,
INCLUDING ACADEMIC MEDICAL CENTERS

Even though only a small portion of the total industrial funding for biomedical R&D supports academic research, fostering linkages between industry and university research has been of great interest to both sectors for a number of years. The history outlined in the preceding section illustrates some of the legislative efforts to foster academic-industry collaboration. At the same time, federal agencies developed new programs to encourage such collaboration, such as NSF's academic-industry cooperative research centers and engineering research centers. There are now a number of state programs organized with the express purpose of facilitating and supporting new alliances. In addition, some universities have developed industry-sponsored cooperative basic research programs (Government-University-Industry Research Roundtable 1986).

Research interactions between academia and industry grew rapidly from the 1920s through the early 1940s. By the end of World War II, a survey by the National Academy of Sciences indicated that more than 300 companies in a wide variety of industries were supporting research in universities by sponsoring fellowships, scholarships, and direct grants-in-aid. Of these firms, nearly 50 were subsidizing more than 270 biomedical research projects at about 70 universities (Ginzberg and Dutka 1989).

In the decades after World War II, connections between academia and industry slowly weakened, reaching a low point in the early 1970s. The most significant factor contributing to this decline was the dramatic increase in the federal government's support for academic research after the war, particularly basic research (see the "History of Changing Support . . ." section). Increased availability of federal research dollars and the educational needs of the "baby boomers" both contributed to a dramatic expansion of higher education in the United States. This expansion encouraged faculty members to train students for academic careers. At the same time, industry cut back on its support for basic research, eroding an important point of contact between academic and industrial scientists (Ginzberg and Dutka 1989).

Both the industrial funding of university research and the number and variety of collaborative arrangements between universities and industry have significantly increased during the 1980s, although it is difficult actually to count the number and variety of cooperative arrangements already in place (Government-University-Industry Research Roundtable 1986). Also, it is important to put corporate funding in perspective. The total is still less than 7 percent of the total health R&D performed by institutions of higher education (U.S. DHHS, PHS 1990).

Nonetheless, most knowledgeable people who have commented on the matter have remarked on the virtual explosion over the past several years in the number and variety of alliances between academia and industry involving qualitative changes in their form (Government-University-Industry Research Roundtable 1986). Industrial support for academic research ranges from small unrestricted gifts and contract research to highly organized cooperative ventures (Bloom and Randolph 1990).

Companies have organized themselves in a variety of ways to fund and participate in alliances with academia. In some cases, industries have formed funding consortia. In others, corporations have been formed with the express purpose of working with and drawing from university research. Some large R&D companies, such as Monsanto and IBM, are involved with programs at several different universities (Government-University-Industry Research Roundtable 1986).

On the other side, individual universities and academic medical centers may be involved in several different types of arrangements at the same time, some with federal funding and some without, some with multiple corporate sponsors and others funded by a single company. Also, several academic institutions may jointly participate in an alliance with industry. A number of specific examples of some the different arrangements within academia may be found in the National Academy of Sciences' Government-University-Industry Research Roundtable (GUIRR) report on *New Alliances and Partnerships in American Science and Engineering* (Government-University-Industry Research Roundtable 1986).

Many issues are involved when cooperative ventures are developed between academic institutions and industry. The partnership activities can vary from those largely concerned with basic research to those intended to solve a well-defined practical problem. In addition, many cooperative efforts are associated with the training of undergraduate or graduate students (Government-University-Industry Research Roundtable 1986).

The goals and expectations of industry and its academic partners also are reflected in the nature of the activities. Some academics simply want to augment funds for specific types of research or to supplement their own income through consulting arrangements. Others believe that better access to corporate R&D enhances their own competence and knowledge or affords better opportunities for their students to find industrial jobs. For their part, the industrial partners are often seeking access to experts in a particular scientific field or wish to develop a particular process or product. This access to academia can help to maintain the scientific vitality of their industry as well as to provide access to a steady supply of well-trained scientists (Government-University-Industry Research Roundtable 1986). Obviously, meshing the goals and expectations of industry and the academy is crucial to the success of any cooperative venture (Bloom and Randolph 1990).

In addition, the organization and governance of academic-industrial partnerships vary widely. Some are located within regular academic departments; others involve separate facilities outside the main academic organization. In some arrangements, corporate sponsors only broadly define fields of inquiry at the time of funding. In others, corporate representatives sit on committees that closely oversee the direction of research, or contracts define the objective quite specifically (Government-University-Industry Research Roundtable 1986).

The GUIRR identified the following five types of partnerships into which the nature of the activities, expectations, and university and industry cultures and governance characteristics tended to be clustered:

1. Research programs or centers that support many research projects, and that are closely tied to general academic research and teaching activities—These tend to support more "basic" research, with specified commercial product or process development not usually being involved.
2. Focused projects involving both a well-defined practical objective and intellectual goals—These often use a research team of both university and corporate scientists.
3. Programs developed to help commercialize faculty research—These programs may develop out of earlier contract arrangements.
4. Programs or institutions organized to help clients, that operate outside the university—The service provided may be directed to industry or a government agency.
5. Free-standing research institutes, linked to several universities— While these organizations depend on part-time participation of university faculty and other university resources, they are designed to operate more like a corporate laboratory or a contract research facility.

The research agreement between Washington University Medical School and Monsanto is an example of the first type of industrial support for university research. Monsanto recognized that nearby Washington University could provide the access to biomedical scientists that Monsanto needed to enter the health care industry. This one-on-one relationship supports research on peptides and proteins that regulate cellular function and communication. The basic function of the program is to allocate research funds provided by Monsanto. An internal review committee composed of equal numbers of Monsanto and Washington University members reviews grant proposals and awards funds in a process very similar to that used by NIH study sections. Scientists may publish research results, provided Monsanto has had 30 days to review the report before it is submitted for publication. Under this arrangement, Monsanto is expected to provide the university with $62 million for research by 1990 (Bloom and Randolph 1990, Government-University-Industry Research Roundtable 1986).

NONPROFIT ORGANIZATIONS SUPPORTING BIOMEDICAL RESEARCH

Private foundations were the main external source of university research funds from the late 1800s to the end of World War II. Most foundations were established to address specified social or health problems or to benefit particular institutions. During the twentieth century, hundreds of voluntary health agencies (also known as "operating foundations") were formed, supported by contributions from constituents or the general public. In addition, a special type of nonprofit organization called the "medical research organization" was created, with the Howard Hughes Medical Institute (HHMI) being the most well-known example (Bloom and Randolph 1990, Boniface and Rimel 1987).

Since World War II, investment in biomedical R&D by industry and the federal government has overshadowed the magnitude of contributions by the nonprofit sector. NIH estimated that private nonprofit organizations contributed about $827 million, or about 4 percent of all support for health R&D, in 1990 (U.S. DHHS, PHS 1990). Although these organizations now contribute a substantially smaller share of the total national investment in biomedical research than they have in the past, they are still considered vital to the nation's research enterprise. They provide another source of funds that is generally more flexible and often is targeted toward preventing and curing specified human diseases. Nonprofit support for biomedical research augments funds available from federal sources and can provide crucial support by filling gaps in the research agenda that—for policy or other reasons—have not been adequately addressed by government or industry (Bloom and Randolph 1990).

There is probably not one nonprofit organization that typifies this group because there is such broad variety among them in their missions, governance, and the ways they provide research support. The following sections review the development and general characteristics of nonprofit organizations that support medical research in this country.

Foundations

Gifts from an individual, family, or company to a foundation provide the financial base from which grant money can be derived. It has been estimated that nearly 400 of the approximately 4000 largest U.S. foundations support some form of biomedical research (Boniface and Rimel 1987). Since the growth in the NIH budget surpassed the combined research budgets of all private foundations a number of years ago, these organizations have generally adopted the role of the "venture capitalist" for supporting research. Common strategies include the support of the first independent efforts of young researchers, and initial investments in emerging research fields.

Health has always been a popular area of activity for private foundations. While a few foundations still conduct some type of in-house research, most have determined that supporting extramural research is the most productive way to use their funds. Foundations support research in a variety of ways, including individual research project grants, fellowships, equipment grants, support for new professorships, and sponsorship of conferences, workshops, or educational programs. Examples of some of the foundations that contribute to biomedical research include the Pew Charitable Trusts, the Lucille P. Markey Trust, the Commonwealth Fund, the Alfred P. Sloan Foundation, the Rockefeller Foundation, and the John D. and Catherine T. MacArthur Foundation (Bloom and Randolph 1990).

Priorities for foundations are determined in a variety of ways. Sometimes, funding decisions are made based on interest in a specified disease or through personal contacts. Smaller foundations may not plan specified programs but fund the best unsolicited proposal received. On the other hand, other foundations may only consider proposals they solicit, and they may use expert advice and a peer-review process similar to that used by the NIH. Company-sponsored foundations may limit their support to projects in particular locations or to programs that directly affect their employees (Bloom and Randolph 1990).

Voluntary Health Agencies

Voluntary health agencies are public charities supported mainly by donations from a constituency or the general public. Many voluntary health agencies were originally founded by family and friends of individuals suffering from a particular disease. Voluntary health agencies are also known as "operating foundations." There are nearly 200 national and regional organizations actively supporting some type of biomedical research. Many of the larger voluntary health agencies have local chapters and a national office. Some of the more well-known voluntary health agencies include the American Cancer Society and the American Heart Association (Bloom and Randolph 1990, Boniface and Rimel 1987).

Voluntary health agencies are involved in a variety of activities, including grants for research and training, public education, patient referrals, and lobbying for increased federal funding related to the diseases or disorders that concern them. Although these organizations often cannot make long-term commitments to research efforts, they are able to provide funds to help researchers launch their careers and to develop novel lines of investigation (Bloom and Randolph 1990). As for foundations, support may come in the form of individual project grants, fellowships, support for new initiatives, or short-term emergency funding (Boniface and Rimel 1987).

The Howard Hughes Medical Institute

The HHMI is a medical research organization (MRO) that was founded in 1953. As an MRO, HHMI must be actively engaged in conducting medical research and must spend 3.5 percent of its endowment on research each year. The HHMI endowment was valued at $5 billion in 1987, and it has become the major private contributor to biomedical research (Bloom and Randolph 1990).

HHMI support for research totaled $209.5 million in 1990, which is comparable to the budget of a small NIH institute. HHMI supports research in immunology, cell biology, genetics, neuroscience, and structural biology. Designed to complement federal funding for research in these areas, HHMI supports selected groups of researchers within universities and hospitals around the country, providing full funding for faculty and technician salaries, as well as paying for all research expenses. In 1990, HHMI employed 208 investigators in about 50 sites nationwide (Bloom and Randolph 1990, Bloom, personal communication, April 1991).

THE FUTURE OF FUNDING FOR BIOMEDICAL RESEARCH

The forecast for the funding of biomedical research in the remainder of this century might be titled "More of the same." The aforementioned trends—a slowing in the rate of growth in government funding, a growth in industry-sponsored research—will generally continue.

For the government, a diminished rate of growth in funding will be the likely result of extreme, competing pressures. On the one hand, the U.S. Congress has traditionally been highly supportive of biomedical research. Cutting-edge research on diseases plays well for political constituencies, and members of Congress often have personal interests in particular diseases. On the other hand, the impetus to cut the budget deficit constrains every area of the federal budget, including funding for science research. The push for large science projects, such as the superconducting supercollider and biomedicine's own Human Genome

Project, will create further competition even within limited agency budgets. Therefore, unless the problem of the budget deficit is resolved or there is a dramatic reordering of priorities in the federal government, the current direction of government funding for biomedicine is unlikely to change in the immediate future.

Industry, on the other hand, is likely to accelerate its search for new products in the dramatically burgeoning field of biomedical science. Industrial research laboratories will probably build their biomedical research staffs, and competition for the limited number of top-notch scientists will push corporations toward funding more cooperative ventures with universities. Nonetheless, though industrial funding of R&D is likely to increase, most of the increase is likely to come in the funding of development and not in basic research. A change in federal tax policy could provide incentives for companies to do more basic research, but because a major change in tax policy would probably come about only with a general agreement on how to address the budget deficit, little change is likely.

The potential implications for the nation are both positive and negative. Because the supply of biomedical researchers is going to grow faster than the supply of money to fund them, those researchers will be forced to compete more fiercely for funding and spend more time on grant applications. Scientists may move from academia to industry in greater numbers.

Universities will also find money harder to come by and may adopt a more conservative approach to science research by choosing to hire scientists with proven track records rather than untried, young scientists with more adventurous theories. There probably also will be a tendency to form umbrella programs in a general subject such as cardiovascular research or cognitive science. Through such specialization, institutions can seek large grants for one program that will support many scientists.

Last, because industrial funding of biomedical research is steadily increasing, universities and individual scientists will naturally strive to form more partnerships with industry. That potential conflicts exist in such collaborations is detailed in much of the rest of this book, but the rewards of such collaborations should be great. The products and technology that scientists create out of basic research will lead to both a stronger and more competitive economy and a healthier society. In summary, although current trends in funding will probably dictate that basic biomedical research will grow more slowly than applied research, this situation has the potential to strengthen the nation and the applied sciences, without posing an immediate threat to the preeminence of the country's basic research in biomedicine.

REFERENCES

Bloom, F., and Randolph, M. Eds. 1990. *Funding Health Sciences Research: A Strategy to Restore Balance.* Washington, D.C.: National Academy Press.

Boniface, Z. E., and Rimel, R. W. 1987. *U.S. Funding of Biomedical Research.* Philadelphia: Pew Charitable Trusts.

Buderi, R., Carey, J. et al. 1991. The brakes go on in R&D. *Business Week,* July 1, pp. 24–26.

Ginzberg E., and Dutka, A. B. 1989. *The Financing of Biomedical Research.* Baltimore: The Johns Hopkins University Press.

Government-University-Industry Research Roundtable, National Academy of Sciences. 1986. *New Alliances and Partnerships in American Science and Engineering.* Washington, D.C.: National Academy Press.

Government-University-Industry Research Roundtable, National Academy of Sciences. 1989. *Science and Technology in the Academic Enterprise: Status, Trends, and Issues.* Washington, D.C.: National Academy Press.

National Science Foundation. 1987. *Biotechnology Research and Development Activities in Industry, 1984 and 1985.* Washington, D.C.: NSF, pp. 87–311.

Office of Management and Budget. 1990. *Budget of the United States Government, Fiscal Year 1991.* Washington, D.C.: U.S. Government Printing Office.

Office of Management and Budget. 1991. *Budget of the United States Government, Fiscal Year 1992.* Washington, D.C.: U.S. Government Printing Office.

Office of Technology Assessment, U.S. Congress. 1984. *Commercial Biotechnology: An International Analysis.* (Document No. OTA-BA-218). Washington, D.C.:

Office of Technology Assessment, U.S. Congress. 1988. *New Developments in Biotechnology: U.S. Investment in Biotechnology* (PB88-246939). Washington, D.C.: National Technical Information Service, U.S. Department of Commerce.

Pharmaceutical Manufacturers Association. 1990. *Annual Survey Report of the U.S. Pharmaceutical Industry, 1988–1990.* Washington, D.C.

U.S. Department of Health and Human Services, Public Health Service. 1990. *NIH Data Book, 1990* (Publication No. 90-1261). Bethesda, Maryland: National Institutes of Health.

3 • The Contribution of Biomedical Science and Technology to U.S. Economic Competitiveness

Christopher C. Vaughan, Bruce L. R. Smith, and Roger J. Porter

Only half a century ago, the concepts of sickness and health were quite different from those of today. Parents generally expected that some of their children would die in infancy, and in the preantibiotic era, it was more or less expected that some of those who made it through infancy would die of infections such as bacterial pneumonia. Death and disability were still relatively common occurrences at all ages. Expectations about health were tempered by discouraging statistics.

In the 1990s, expectations are strikingly different. The loss of a child is uniformly tragic and unexpected. Death in middle age is similarly distressing. The vast majority of us live a healthy life and expect to do so into old age, rather naïvely fearing only accidents in our youth, and cancer and vascular disease as we get older. We expect that children will be born healthy, that infections will disappear with antibiotic treatment, and that artificial hips, heart valves, and knees will replace our natural parts if needed. In short, the expectations for wellness are remarkably higher than was possible or reasonable fifty years ago.

The reasons for this change are complex and include improved sanitation, antibiotics, life-style changes, antihypertensive medications, and much more. The causes, however, are not what is emphasized here; rather, we emphasize the *impact* of this shift in expectations on medicine and medical research, the financial impact of health research, and most especially, the competitive implications of the health care revolution in the United States. The aim is to assess how the United States can maintain a continuous improvement in health care with advanced technology and sustain the American position as world leader in research and development of those technologies.

SPENDING FOR HEALTH CARE IN THE UNITED STATES

The desire for wellness has been a major force in bringing about improvements in the quality and effectiveness of medicine during this century. However, a healthier society has come at a price. Americans spend more per capita on health care than any other industrialized nation (Figure 3.1). As a nation, the United States also spends more of its gross national product (GNP), or wealth, on health care than other industrialized nations; an estimated $647 billion, or 12 percent of its GNP, was allocated to health care in 1990 (Gladwell 1991). This high cost, along with the problems of the uninsured, has led to a crisis in health care that has reawakened the debate on the reform of health care financing.

The United States did not always pay so much for medical goods and services. In 1965, the nation spent only 6.0 percent of the GNP on health care. Even as the GNP grew since the mid-1960s, however, the amount spent on health grew more rapidly, consuming on average an additional 1 percent of the GNP every five years.

Figure 3.1. The per capita spending on health (in U.S. dollars) and the percentage of the gross domestic product spent on health in 1986 in countries belonging to the Organization for Economic Cooperation and Development.

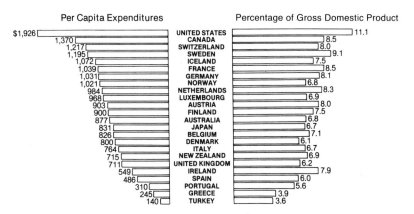

Source: Ryan, T.J. et al., 1990. Reprinted with permission from the American College of Cardiology (*Journal of the American College of Cardiology* 16, no. 1 [1990]).

The United States may have the most expensive medical care, but it is not alone in watching costs rise. Other nations have also seen a constant elevation in the price of health care in relation to their GNP. These figures reinforce an argument supported by common sense: The desire for wellness exists throughout the world, and where the technology, education, and a strong economy make it possible to satisfy that desire, people will spend money on health care.

The extraordinary growth of the medical industry has been paradoxical in its effect, making medical technology not only a powerful and important sector of the economy but also a potential drain on the GNP. In 1989, the U.S. manufacturers of health-care products (other than pharmaceuticals produced $28.7 billion in products. The 1989 sales figures are 10 percent higher than the previous year, and 1990 sales are estimated to show another 9 percent rise to $31.2 billion (Health Industry Manufacturers Association 1991). When compared to the $10.5 billion of medical devices and diagnostics produced in 1980, it is obvious that the medical products sector has been one of the economy's fastest growing during the 1980s. In fact, of the six industrial sectors projected by the U.S. Department of Commerce to be the fastest growing in 1991, three were from the health-technology industry: surgical and medical instruments (forecast to grow 9%), surgical appliances and supplies (8%), and diagnostic substances (7%) (Health Industry Manufacturers Association 1991).

Equally impressive, and related to the same dynamic, is the growth of pharmaceutical manufacturing in the United States. The U.S. Pharmaceutical Manufacturers Association (PMA), a trade association representing most American, research-based, pharmaceutical manufacturers, reports that U.S. sales of member companies grew from $11.8 billion in 1980 to an estimated $36.2 billion in 1990 (PMA 1991).

The fuel for this growth has been partly the reimbursement mechanisms that pay for the results of technological progress. Payments from the federal government account for a sizable fraction of what consumers expend for health care, hence prompting the critics of what is often called the "health-industrial complex" to complain that public expenditures, and not market forces, produce the dynamic growth of the medical technology and pharmaceutical industries.

Despite the accuracy of many of these criticisms, the portion of the nation's wealth allocated to health care is unlikely to diminish over the next quarter century, and will probably increase (Aaron 1991). The thirst for first-class health care will not go away; further, the population of the United States is aging rapidly. If demography is destiny, then the economic destiny of the United States is to become a nation that devotes a large and perhaps still-growing percentage of its GNP to support a large elderly population requiring increasing medical care. The public has already manifested its expectations about the medical care it will tolerate and aspire to. Americans want the best care, and they want it now.

Higher deductibles and copayments have not noticeably slowed the growth of costs. A much slower rate of growth in medical spending has been achieved in Great Britain through their National Health Service, but important differences between the United Kingdom and the United States indicate that the British program would not work here (Aaron and Schwartz 1984, Ryan et al. 1990). Rationing or implicit rationing in the Medicaid system has generated a storm of criticism and therefore would be difficult to pursue in the United States. The effort by Oregon to seek a waiver to reform its Medicaid system illustrates the problems of such an approach. Oregon eventually was forced to restore coverage for categories of transplant surgery it had sought to exclude from Medicaid reimbursement.

The treatment of the terminally ill, such as those with AIDS, is a good example of the cutting edge of the phenomenon of escalating costs. The AIDS epidemic has forced the U.S. government to change the approval process for new drugs so that patients can get them sooner, and AIDS patients are putting pressure on insurance companies to pay for expensive drugs that a decade ago would have been classified as "experimental" and therefore not covered by insurance. People with chronic disorders, following the same path, now ask why they cannot get new treatments immediately and at minimal cost to themselves. For these reasons and others, the Health Care Financing Administration (HCFA) of the U.S. Department of Health and Human Services estimated in 1990 that by the year 2000, the nation will dedicate a full 15 percent of the GNP to health care (Figure 3.2). This figure may yet be revised upward. In fact, after this estimate was made, the preliminary figures for health care expenditures in 1990 were tabulated and found to be .2 percent of GNP more than projected under the HCF scenario—for a total of 12.2 percent of GNP (Gladwell 1991).

Political pressures to contain this rapid rise in costs are increasingly being felt in the U.S. Congress and in the executive branch, as well as in the private sector. The size of the nation's health care bill and its rate of growth are such that reforms intended to regulate pricing and limit cost increases may be inevitable in the next few years. However, such measures seem destined only to slow, and not stop, the growth in health costs. As the nation seeks to control medical costs, measures that reduce access to some medical treatments will evoke an

Figure 3.2. The costs of health care as a percentage of the GNP.

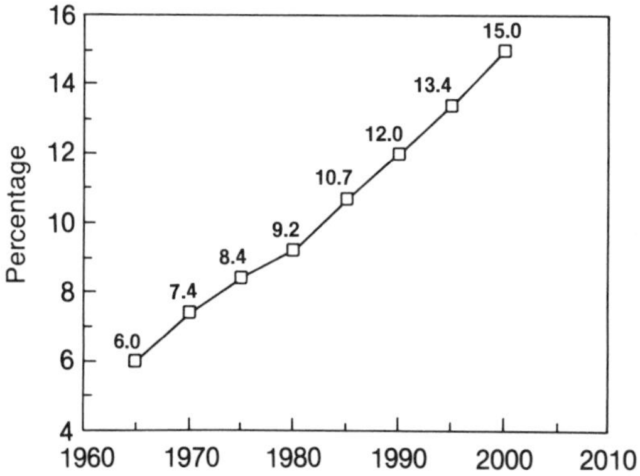

Source: Data from Ryan, T.J. et al., 1990; HCFA. Reprinted with permission from the American College of Cardiology (*Journal of the American College of Cardiology* 16, no. 1 [1990]: 18).
Note: Years 1990–2000 are estimates.

opposing political pressure to spend the money necessary to provide the medical care that people expect. There is little reason to expect health care costs to decrease markedly despite strenuous cost-containment efforts. The dynamic is ultimately driven by the expectation not only of health but also of rapid cure when disease does strike. The operative forces are deeply rooted in cultural attitudes and values, not in mechanical features of the health care financing system or administrative practices. For cost control to be realized, expectations about rights and entitlements will have to change.

THE FUTURE OF THE BIOMEDICAL INDUSTRY

External Constraints on Growth

Strong domestic medical technology and pharmaceutical industries are important for the balance of trade and for a strong economy generally. As the MIT Commission on Industrial Productivity concludes, in its authoritative study *Made in America* (Dertouzos, Lester, and Solow 1989), when Americans have technological leadership, they also retain economic leadership. However, the authors also note that prowess in basic science does not necessarily lead to technological leadership: "The United States is still unarguably the leader in basic research. The scale of its scientific enterprise is unequaled, and it is second to none in making new discoveries. Yet U.S. companies increasingly find themselves lagging behind their foreign rivals in the commercial exploitation of inventions and discoveries . . . even though the enabling technological advances were first made in the U.S." (Dertouzos, Lester, and Solow 1989).

The billions in products that are currently produced in the United States to satisfy U.S. demand could as easily be produced in other industrialized nations. If we do not produce them, others will probably do so. The trade deficit could thus be exacerbated if the United States were to lose its technological edge in medical devices and biomedicine. *Such a situation would give us the worst of both worlds: escalating health care costs* and *dependence on foreign sources of supply.* This would be particularly tragic because the United States currently holds so many strengths in biomedicine, such as a strong research base and extensive experience in biomedical manufacturing. Nonetheless, can the United States continue to enjoy a dominant position? To protect and foster American strengths, we must understand the factors that can detrimentally affect this important industry.

Among the factors that potentially constrain the U.S. biomedical industry, the failure to invest sufficiently in research and development (R&D) is a major concern. Even though the pharmaceutical industry is among the highest in R&D as a percentage of sales (14–16%), much of the investment is directed toward exploiting current lines of technology and product development (Vagelos 1991). The transition to new products, in particular the development of products based on the new biogenetics, is a critical challenge for the industry. The rising development costs for new products that genuinely push out the technological frontier by substantially improving on former products increase the risks associated with innovation and pose a serious threat to the industry (Kline and Rosenberg 1986).

Political efforts to control prices may make some areas of R&D appear unprofitable. There is already some public discontent, for instance, over the pricing of AIDS drugs and resultant talk of taking steps to lower prices. Companies that feel they may be delayed in recouping development costs may decide not to compete in some areas. In political terms, the drug companies are the most inviting targets imaginable. Almost no politician—even some of those with companies in their districts—feels inclined to support the drug industry. The pharmaceutical and medical-device industries are favorite whipping boys, in part because they are chronically suspected of exploiting monopolistic advantages in pricing policy.

Even more important, perhaps, tax policies and the cost of capital affect the pace of innovation in the drug industry. As one of the founders of Genentech pointed out, the availability of venture capital has been instrumental in the founding of new biotechnology firms in the United States (Swanson 1986). Many business executives, especially those in companies that invest a large percentage of profits back into research, complain that they are injured by tax laws that limit the research costs they can deduct. The high cost of capital in the United States also discourages R&D and may promote short-term over long-term business strategy. If, for example, a Japanese company borrows $1 million to develop a new product at a real cost of 1.5 percent per year, the company must plan to make more than $100,000 eight years later when the product is marketed in order to pay back the loan. If a U.S. company borrows $1 million at 6 percent real interest, it must plan to make more than $300,000 eight years later in order to cover the capital costs (Hatsopoulous, Krugman, and Summers 1988). Further, the Japanese company, given eight years to increase its investment capital by one tenth, might more easily decide that such a venture carries low risk. A U.S. company, using discounted cash-flow analysis and faced with a similar challenge, to make a profit, might decide that its need to increase the initial investment is too high a risk. Clearly, low capital costs can be a critical competitive advantage.

In addition to financial considerations, regulations can be a constraint on any industry. Because people's health is potentially at risk, the biomedical industry will inevitably be strongly regulated. While companies have generally learned to live with those regulations, the rising cost of medical care is likely to invite more economic controls. Business leaders, in particular, are concerned about the effects of legislation that would seek to control matters such as drug pricing. Public sensitivity to the perceived dangers of recombinant deoxyribonucleic acid (DNA) research has also led to regulations that, in the opinion of scientists as well as industrialists, unnecessarily stifle biotechnology research (Watson 1986). Further, how regulations are administered is critical to their effectiveness. Even when reasonable regulations are in place, the necessary adjunct to any set of regulations—the implementing machinery—may be cumbersome, inefficient, or worse. One of the primary concerns of business leaders is that the Food and Drug Administration (FDA) remains understaffed and slow to act (Swanson 1986). The Patent and Trademark Office (PTO) is also understaffed and has long had a large backlog of biotechnology patents waiting to be examined (Goldhammer 1991).

On the international scene, trade barriers can and do inhibit companies trying to establish new markets for a product. Such barriers range from incongruent regulatory standards among countries to outright limitations on imported products and absence of protection for intellectual property rights. In some countries, the outright thievery of intellectual property due to weak patent laws or a lack of enforcement is an insurmountable problem for industry. American pharmaceutical companies have given up doing any business in Argentina, for instance. In Brazil, the situation is also serious because even drugs protected by U.S. patents can be manufactured and freely sold by any Brazilian company.

Internal Constraints: Managerial Attitudes Toward Innovation

Biomedical research and the medical technology and pharmaceutical industries are more closely linked than are research and applications in virtually any other part of the nation's economy. All of the aforementioned constraints are external to the biomedical business or research center, but there are also constraining factors that can exist inside organizations. Ultimately, these internal variables may be the most important determinants of the future health of the whole industry. An overly conservative approach to new projects among industrial managers can stifle creativity and block new ventures. A conservative attitude on the part of university administrators can similarly discourage faculty interaction with industry.

Creative ideas, of course, require the continuous infusion of new talent and adequate levels of research support. Conservatism can impede innovation at many stages in the product-realization process, but conservatism in research is the most severe impediment. It can doom the potential development of new products from the outset. If there is nothing in the pipeline, the downstream decisions will be limited to exploiting the last bit of advantage from existing product lines (Vagelos 1991). This linkage between research and applications is so critical that it merits separate analysis.

THE CRITICAL ROLE OF RESEARCH IN THE
BIOMEDICAL INDUSTRY

Technology has been *the* driving force in the long-term economic growth of industrial societies, and as technological innovations have become more complex, they have relied more and more on the methodology and findings of scientific research (Landau and Rosenberg 1986). Perhaps more than in other industries, such research is the core and driving force of the biomedical industry. The postwar consensus on science policy emphasized the importance of research as the linch-pin of industrial development in all sectors of the economy (Smith 1991), but the biomedical area most clearly illustrates the pattern of academic research leading directly to commercialization. The United States is the leader in biotechnology today because the country has invested enormous sums in research since World War II (Swanson 1986).

Now, more than ever before, technological advances in biomedi-cine begin in science. The quality and speed of discovery has become more and more important in getting patents on inventions and moving products to market. The distinction between basic and applied research has blurred as the time between discovery and product development has shortened.

The pace of scientific advancement and the nature of the industry demand intensive efforts in research. A generic drug, notwithstanding the recent scandals involving fraud in the FDA, may be nearly as good as the name brand and can be sold at a much lower price. The advan-tage of the company producing the generic drug stems from the fact that the company does not have to recoup the cost of research, devel-opment, and clinical trials. For that reason, most pharmaceutical com-panies must depend mainly on profits from those drugs still under pat-ent protection and must therefore have a constant supply of new products in the pipeline.

Although companies benefit from collaborations with universities and academic medical centers, the pharmaceutical companies them-selves sponsor research on a large scale (Vagelos 1991) (Figure 3.3). The need for continuous innovation is also present in the medical tech-

Figure 3.3. The price index of Merck medicines (dotted line), the consumer price index (CPI) (dashed line), and Merck's spending on R&D (solid line).

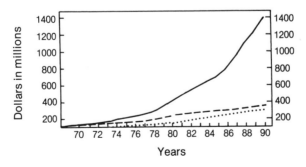

Source: Vagelos 1991. Copyright 1991 by the AAAS.
Note: The variable represented by each line starts at an index level of 100 in 1969.

nology and diagnostic industries. As noted in a 1990 survey by the Health Industry Manufacturers Association, the U.S. health-care technology industry invested 6.2 percent of sales in R&D, thereby outinvesting other research-intensive industries such as aerospace (4.1 percent of sales invested in R&D), chemicals (3.8 percent), and electrical and electronics (5.4 percent) (Health Industry Manufacturers Association 1991). The level of R&D in the pharmaceutical industry is even greater. In 1990, the 89 member companies of the PMA invested over $8 billion in R&D, a figure that represented an estimated 16.8 percent of sales for the industry (Pharmaceutical Manufacturers Association 1991). This money is generally well spent. Studies of the economies of scale in biomedical research indicate that more spending on R&D does produce more new products (Schwartzman 1975).

Because research plays such an important role in the success or failure of biomedicine, the health of the research enterprise deserves close examination. Research can be stifled at the most fundamental level if the supply of talented researchers or the quality of their advanced training in the universities weakens. A company cannot generate good ideas without well-trained scientists; the universities will continue to be crucial in this respect. The fertility of the company milieu, in turn, is important and will depend on a number of factors. Modern biological science demands highly advanced equipment of the type that used to be the province of physicists or chemists. Ultracentrifuges that spin at a rate of 60,000 revolutions per minute (rpm) are standard. DNA and protein sequencers and peptide synthesizers are required for much of the biotechnology work. Gas chromatographs and mass spectrographs are a requirement for chemical analysis.

Funds must also be available for expensive supporting services (Vagelos 1991). Scientists need to run expensive assays and use expensive enzymes when necessary. Access to on-line databases are a necessity of modern laboratories. Companies also must be willing to pay for services such as DNA cloning and amplification by an outside company. Scientists must also be assisted by properly trained research assistants who can perform complex procedures reliably.

In addition to all these factors, scientists need broad management support to combat unnecessary red tape. A certain degree of insulation from the normal cares of the company can help scientists exert their best efforts in the laboratory.

Shortages of trained scientists are already a problem for some companies; the difficulty is expected to worsen (National Research Council [NRC] 1989). Particularly worrisome for biomedical companies are shortages of specialists such as pharmacologists, enzymologists, and toxicologists. A 1989 survey published by the NRC showed

Table 3.1. Occupational Employment in Dedicated Biotechnology Companies, 1989

Occupation	Total Employed	Total Ph.D.s Employed	Shortage as a Percentage of Employed	Planned Hires as a Percentage of Employed
Molecular genetics	724	340	2.7	13.8
Classical genetics	42	20	5.1	15.3
Industrial microbiology	311	72	9.8	29.3
General microbiology	665	248	1.2	10.1
Human/ animal cell biology	471	198	3.0	10.1
Plant cell biology	86	45	4.5	13.4
Human/ animal molecular biology	508	309	9.7	21.7
Plant molecular biology	90	55	3.7	11.1
Human/ animal biology	246	87	3.4	11.5
Plant biology	42	25	4.0	15.8
Pharmacology	209	93	11.9	25.9
Toxicology	73	17	17.8	29.7
Enzymology	81	59	11.9	27.2
Immunology	532	216	7.9	20.8
Other biology	154	39	2.5	15.3
Analytical biochemistry	377	156	3.9	20.5
General biochemistry	1042	498	6.0	17.7
Other chemistry	1397	644	5.0	21.7
Other biotechnology specialties	369	163	3.7	43.0
Total	7420	3282	5.4	19.4

Source: National Research Council, 1989.

shortages of these specialists in the double digits as a percentage of those employed (Table 3.1).

BIOTECHNOLOGY: THE NEW FRONTIER

Much has been made of the opportunities in molecular biology. The increased ability to locate genes and to sequence DNA codes has caught the popular imagination because these genes determine whether a person has brown eyes, is short or tall, dies young from muscular dystrophy, or suffers familial Alzheimer's disease. Nonetheless, most of the larger American pharmaceutical companies have yet to invest fully in this arena because it is new and expensive, its potential seems uncertain, and it requires a longer-term investment than many companies can afford. Pharmaceutical companies in the United States are enjoying a relatively high state of productivity and profitability, and they are content to pursue older, more proven research directions rather than invest in new ones. Further, the industry has been apathetic because of the slowness of scientific advances in biotechnology, both in the identification of genes and the creation of some workable theses for utilizing genetic information in therapeutic efforts. This lethargic approach is almost certainly a grave mistake.

The Scientific Potential of Biotechnology

First, the potential benefits of biotechnology are exceptionally large. Each new biotechnology product can be uniquely tailored to a specific problem because the mechanism that is targeted is so fundamental. There is nothing that could so profoundly alter medical practice than the ability to alter the genetic code. Not only is the new generation of genetically engineered drugs highly specific, but these drugs' toxicity may also prove to be a smaller obstacle to their development and approval than hitherto believed. The brain alone uses the products of approximately 30,000 genes. Although the vast majority of these genes may not be involved in disease, the understanding of those that *are* important is the next frontier of neuroscience.

Biotechnology's Vast Economic Potential

The drugs that *have* been developed are high value-added products—that is, they are frequently very expensive but are highly efficacious. An example is *erythropoietin,* which stimulates the production of red blood cells. The drug may be needed by as many as 50,000 patients with renal failure. At a per-patient cost of $4,500 per year, the potential gross revenues from this drug are as high as $280 million (Thompson 1991). Worldwide, approximately 175,000 patients may be candidates for the drug (Miskell 1986). This is just one drug for one small part of the patient population. What is the value of drugs for more common diseases? The 1980s was a decade of watching and waiting, but the 1990s should be a decade of action.

The Logarithmic Pace of Progress in Gene Identification

Most scientists agree that only about 3 percent of the human genome contains meaningful information; the rest is, as far as we know, silent and not of major scientific interest. The search for genes using standard techniques was relatively slow until National Institute of Neurological Disorders and Stroke scientist Craig Venter and his colleagues found the meaningful part of the DNA. Using human brain complementary DNA (cDNA) derived from RNA (ribonucleic acid, the chain derived from DNA), these investigators reported the discovery of 337 new human genes in the brain (Adams et al. 1991). This cDNA-sequencing technique may provide the basis for identification by 1994 of virtually all of the genes that encode the human brain and of all human genes by 1996. Every one of these genes is potentially patentable. Even if this estimate is optimistic, and even if we do not yet know the utility, if any, of most of the genes that have been sequenced by this method, the opportunities are suddenly much closer than was previously imagined. These discoveries illustrate the fast-paced movement of this field and the potential for wholly new products yielding great profitability.

Existing Pragmatic Strategies for Gene Therapies

One of the pragmatic strategies now available is the concept of *antisense RNA*. If RNA is the message, and if the message derived from defective DNA is erroneous, the development by molecular biology of an RNA that is antisense and that will negate the action of the defective RNA (by blocking the production of a defective protein) is a logical therapeutic approach (Melton 1985). Another possible therapeutic approach is the *triple-helix formation,* in which the defective DNA on the chromosome is identified and negated (Maher, Wold, and Dervan 1989). Both approaches require knowledge of the exact DNA or RNA sequence to be silenced, but once these sequences are known, the construction of the oligonucleotide that will be effective may prove surprisingly easy. We are only seeing the first of many exciting avenues

Figure 3.4. Biotechnology companies and products in the United States and Japan, 1989.

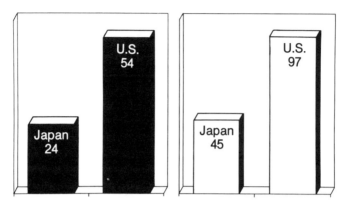

Source: Pharmaceutical Manufacturers Association, 1989.

for using genetic information to prevent or cure disease (Weatherall 1991). The existing therapeutic product base could be swept aside by an avalanche of newer and more effective products.

In Jeopardy: U.S. Leadership in Biotechnology

The United States is the current leader in biotechnology, but it could lose its lead rapidly. Although others are beginning to close the gap, the United States is still the undisputed leader in R&D. The United States has, for example, a two-to-one advantage over Japan in the number of biotechnology companies and in the number of products approved or under development (Figure 3.4). Nonetheless, this lead is hardly cause for complacency. The biotechnology industry shows a pattern familiar to other U.S. industries—a failure to translate a technological edge in the laboratory into products. If the United States does not enjoy early success with the new products of biotechnology, the profits that make possible further research may erode, and a new dynamic in the industry could be created.

BIOMEDICINE IN THE INTERNATIONAL MARKETPLACE

How important is technological leadership in biomedicine to the U.S. economy? In 1989, the United States exported $5.5 billion and imported $3.1 billion in medical equipment and diagnostics, generating a trade surplus of $2.3 billion. For the period 1990–95, the spread between imports and exports of these products is predicted to grow at an annual rate of nearly 25 percent and to provide an $8.4 billion trade surplus by 1995 (PMA 1991). The U.S. pharmaceutical industry also contributes to a surplus in the area of trade. In 1988, the industry exported $3.9 billion in pharmaceutical products, and the country imported $3.6 billion in pharmaceuticals, leaving a positive balance of trade of $300 million in this area.

More important, perhaps, is the fact that, in 1990, U.S. drug companies manufactured abroad more than $20 billion in pharmaceuticals. Those drugs manufactured abroad are also mostly sold abroad, but the United States benefits from the strong posture of American companies overseas. Dividends flowing back to American shareholders are only one indicator of this broad benefit. Even though sales of U.S. companies abroad do not show up as exports on the U.S. payments balance, they are of obvious importance for the overall vitality of the American pharmaceutical industry.

There are signs, though, that the United States is losing its leading position in biomedicine. As evidence of this, N. Bruce Hannay cited a 50 percent decline, since 1970, in the U.S. share of world pharmaceutical R&D expenditures, and a 50 percent decline in the number of U.S.-owned drugs entering clinical trials during the same period (Hannay 1986).

Of course, many European or Japanese companies similarly manufacture and sell products in the United States. This raises the question of what is a "U.S." company. In an increasingly international economy, does it matter whether the companies that manufacture products in the United States and generate jobs here are American companies legally? What, indeed, constitutes a definition of American versus foreign ownership?

CORPORATE NATIONALITY: WHO BENEFITS?

In 1990, the Swiss company Roche Holding Ltd., parent company to the drug firm Hoffmann–LaRoche, bought a controlling interest in the genetic engineering company Genentech, shaking up the industry and the biotechnology stock indexes. That a pharmaceutical firm had bought a biotechnology company was no surprise—such acquisitions had been going on for years, as cash-short research boutiques merged with large firms that had strong manufacturing capability and the capital to commercialize the smaller firm's inventions. What surprised the American public was that a non-U.S. drug company had bought the first, the largest, and seemingly the only successful genetic engineering company to date in the nation. Genentech's outlook has been clouded, however, with its most successful product—the clot-dissolving drug TPA (tissue plasminogen activator)—coming up against competition from cheaper and safer products.

A superficial view would depict the United States as losing a great asset and the flagship of the industry, but in many important respects, nothing has actually changed much at Genentech after the acquisition. The firm is still based in San Francisco. Employment remains at its former levels. The firm continues to manufacture insulin and other genetically engineered products. In numerous ways, the company is better off because it has the cash to pursue its plans. This cash infusion has allowed the company to do better what it had done before and has allowed managers to plan for the long term (McHarry 1991).

The flow of capital across borders and the interlacing lines of ownership and control have become enormously complicated. The answer to the question of what is best for the United States in this circumstance is no longer straightforward. In analyzing the question of benefit and loss to a country, the matter has to be viewed in four parts: the effects on jobs, profits, taxes, and control. (1) *Jobs*—Jobs are often thought of as the central issue in any public discussion of foreign investment. Jobs for Americans in a foreign-owned but U.S.-based company give Americans a higher standard of living, and their income taxes contribute to the country's tax base. Important questions to ask are, Are American citizens employed by the company? Do American employees hold positions of high authority or only hold low- or mid-level positions? Is R&D, as well as manufacturing and distribution, done in the United States? (2) *Profits*—To what extent do profits flow out of the host country? Do they go to American shareholders and/or foreign shareholders? Are the profits reinvested in new facilities, equipment, and employee training in the United States? (3) *Taxes*—Does the host country get tax income from the foreign-owned company, or are taxes evaded through manipulation or accounting subterfuge? What is considered fair taxation on a multinational company? (4) *Control*— Who controls the fate of the company and its employees? Does the company seek political influence or violate accepted norms of ethical conduct in the host country? Are decisions affecting American workers made only by foreign nationals?

When viewed in these terms, the question of nationality can be seen in clearer perspective. If there is little distinction in these four areas between so-called foreign and American companies, then neither is inherently better for the nation than the other. In fact, foreign ownership often benefits the United States and its citizens. As Robert Reich remarked, corporations will behave in their own best interests: "American corporate executives do worry about the strength of the American economy, but only insofar as the American market is a source of their corporate revenues—and in this respect they are no different from the executives of foreign-owned firms who sell their goods in the American market" (Reich 1991).

There is no simple yardstick or recipe for judging whether a particular purchase or investment by a foreign firm is good for U.S. citizens. Foreign ownership or investment will almost always benefit some Americans, even if it may cost the jobs of, or otherwise hurt, other Americans. Nonetheless, U.S. ownership of foreign assets must not be overlooked. Indeed, the free flow of capital in recent decades has enormously benefited U.S. commercial and financial interests. The United States stands to lose more than it could gain from a slowdown in world trade or a closing of investment opportunities worldwide. The nation should continue to press for a more open world trading system and for the protection of its intellectual property rights.

In the end, the strengths that the United States or any other industrialized nation enjoys will lie in its scientific and technical skills. The most important factor, then, for the nation is to protect the strength of U.S. research institutions and the productivity of its scientists. As long as Americans monopolize science and technology, the country will continue to enjoy a strong position in trade and commerce in biomedical goods and services.

SUMMARY

What can be said to summarize the contribution to date of biomedical science and technology to the competitiveness of the United States? Also, what are the future implications of the fast-paced biomedical developments that are potentially changing the face of the industry? Clearly, the desire for wellness runs very deep, and the willingness of the taxpayer to pay for health (and health research) is substantial. The demand for health involves not only care at the highest levels currently available but also research to provide a likelihood of even better care in the future. The expectation that government will provide this health is not quite universal, but it is increasing dramatically in those countries, including the United States, where a comprehensive system of health care finance is not yet the dominant force. The issue, inevitably, has increasing political impact. Assuming a continued cooling of international tensions, there is every reason to expect that health-care costs will become an increasingly dominant public and private expense in the next century, if not before.

When money is spent, money is made. The biomedical industry is advancing the state of health care by responding vigorously to both scientific and market opportunities. If we assume that expensive, new products will be available, and health costs will not be significantly reduced, the only prudent course for the nation is to maintain a strong base of federal research and technology. We must adopt policies that will help avoid the double-whammy of both paying for highly expensive health care *and* paying those costs in the form of profits to foreign companies.

The United States is, fortunately, in a position to benefit from this new international competition. We currently have the most highly developed biomedical research enterprise, many technological advantages, and a healthy biomedical industry. The opportunity is enormous if we can maintain an open trading system, free movement of capital and technology, and protection of intellectual property rights.

However, the United States also faces considerable risks. Complacency can lead to a loss of our current advantage; other countries understand the stakes of this contest and are gaining ground. For the U.S. biomedical industry to maintain its lead, it must be sensitive to the new dynamics of biomedical product development, recognizing that (1) the milking of current products without investment in the future is suicidal, (2) no lead can be considered comfortable with the dynamic technology of today's highly competitive environment, (3) the trend toward increasing research investment by all companies and increasing capital costs of research is here to stay, (4) protectionism is not the wave of the future and is a counterproductive means to solve the problems of industrial indolence, and (5) risks in new fields of research are unavoidable. Special attention must be given to developments in the new biotechnology, which will soon be a dominant force in biomedical research, technological development, and product sales.

The 1990s are an exciting time for biomedical research. The opportunities for improving health are linked to the promising economics of new product development. These opportunities are closer than most can imagine. The exploitation of both economic and scientific opportunities are essential to the nation and to the fuller life sought by all.

REFERENCES

Aaron, H. J. 1991. *Serious and Unstable Condition: Financing America's Health Care.* Washington, D.C.: Brookings Institution.

Aaron, H. J., and Schwartz, W. B. 1984. *The Painful Prescription: Rationing Medical Care.* Washington, D.C.: Brookings Institution.

Adams, M. D. et al. 1991. Complementary DNA sequencing: Expressed sequence tags and Human Genome Project. *Science,* 252(5013):1651–6.

Dertouzos, M. L., Lester, R. K., and Solow, R. M. 1989. *Made in America.* Cambridge, Massachusetts: MIT Press, pp. 15, 65.

Gladwell, M. 1991. Health costs' share of GNP up sharply. *Washington Post,* April 23, p. 8.

Goldhammer, A. 1991. Spokesperson for the Industrial Biotechnology Association. Personal communication, June.

Hannay, N. B. 1986. Technology and trade: A study of U.S. competitiveness in seven industries. In *The Positive Sum Strategy.* Washington, D.C.: National Academy Press, p. 489.

Hatsopoulous, G. N., Krugman, P. R., and Summers, L. H. 1988. U.S. competitiveness: Beyond the trade deficit. *Science,* 241 (4863): 299–307.

Health Care Financing Administration. 1991. Personal communication with HCFA spokesperson, June.

Health Industry Manufacturers Association. 1991. *Competitiveness of the U.S. Health Care Technology Industry: Contributions to the U.S. Economy and Trade.* Washington, D.C.

Kline, S. J., and Rosenberg, N. 1986. An overview of innovation. In *The Positive Sum Strategy.* Washington, D.C.: National Academy Press, pp. 275–305.

Landau, R., and Rosenberg, N. 1986. *The Positive Sum Strategy.* Washington, D.C.: National Academy Press, p. vi.

Maher, L. J. III, Wold, B., and Dervan, P. B. 1989. Inhibition of DNA binding proteins by oligonucleotide-directed triple helix formation. *Science,* 245 (4919): 725–30.

McHarry, M. 1991. Spokesperson for Genentech. *Personal Communication,* June.

Melton, D. A. 1985. Injected anti-sense RNAs specifically block messenger RNA translation in vivo. *Proceedings of the National Academy of Science,* 82:144–8.

Miskell, J. 1986. *Applied Genetics News.* Stamford, Connecticut: BBC, Inc. 7(2): p. 1.

National Research Council. 1989. *Vol. 1. Biomedical and behavioral research scientists: Their Training and Supply.* Washington, D.C.: National Academy Press.

Pharmaceutical Manufacturers Association. 1989.

Pharmaceutical Manufacturers Association. 1991. *Reporter's Handbook.* Washington, D.C.: PMA.

Reich, R. B. 1991. *The Work of Nations.* New York: Alfred A. Knopf. p. 141.

Ryan, T. J. et al. 1990. Task Force III: Perspectives on the allocation of limited resources in cardiovascular medicine. *Journal of the American College of Cardiology,* 16(1):1–36.

Schwartzman, D. 1975. *The Expected Return from Pharmaceutical Research.* Washington, D.C.: American Enterprise Institute for Public Policy Research.

Smith, B. L. R. 1991. *American Science Policy Since World War II.* Washington, D.C.: Brookings Institution.

Swanson, R. A. 1986. Entrepreneurship and innovation: Biotechnology. In *The Positive Sum Strategy.* Washington, D.C.: National Academy Press. pp. 429–35.

Thompson, L. 1991. The high cost of rare diseases. *Washington Post Health.* June 25, p. 10.

Vagelos, P. R. 1991. Are prescription drug prices high? *Science,* 252 (5010):1080–4.

Watson, J. 1986. From understanding to manipulating DNA. In *The Positive Sum Strategy.* Washington, D.C.: National Academy Press. pp. 213–25.

Weatherall, D. J. 1991. Gene therapy in perspective. *Nature,* 349(6307):275–6.

PART II

The University Medical Center's Outward View of the World and of Industry

4 • The Role and Mission of the University

Hans Mark and Sheldon Ekland-Olson

Universities have been important contributors to Western civilization for 900 years. At the end of the first millennium, groups of clerics assembled in the larger cities in western Europe and established institutions in which people could acquire knowledge in the four classic disciplines: philosophy, medicine, law, and theology. In addition, these institutions took on a broader and perhaps a more important purpose—to provide a common understanding of civilization. This purpose was to be pursued with unshakable faith in two grounding principles: Knowledge is better than ignorance, and some knowledge comes closer to the truth than other knowledge.

While the concept of common understanding is difficult to describe precisely, there is no doubt that it involves something real. Perhaps the best way to illustrate what it has come to mean is by telling a story. Some years ago, when Indira Gandhi was still alive and serving as Prime Minister of India, she entertained British Prime Minister Margaret Thatcher, who was in India for a visit. The two women had a lengthy conversation, and after their meeting, there was the inevitable press conference. One of the reporters asked about the subject of their conversation, to which Mrs. Gandhi replied that it was simply a matter of two old Oxford students getting together and talking about old times at the university. What this story illustrates is that these two distinguished world leaders came away from Oxford University with a perspective on the world, a common understanding of civilization. *Common* does not imply mundane, nor does it mean a lack of appreciation for diversity. It does imply a deep respect for and knowledge of what makes us all human. It is this perspective, knowledge, and respect that allowed these world leaders to transcend their otherwise quite different backgrounds. Mrs. Thatcher came from a lower-middle-class background in central England, and Mrs. Gandhi was a member of the most distinguished aristocratic family in India. Yet somehow the university prepared both of them to assume positions of world leadership. Both of them were able to develop their individual talents and then to acquire the common understanding so necessary for leadership.

The story deals with Oxford University, but a number of other institutions in the world play the same role: the Ecole Normale Superieur and the Ecole Polytechnique in France; the great universities in the cities of Germany; the great private institutions in the United States, such as Harvard and Cornell, and perhaps more important the extensive public university systems that grew from the Homestead Act of 1862. In more recent times, the imperial universities in Japan—the University of Tokyo and the University of Kyoto being the leading ones—have prepared four generations of Japanese to maintain the status of that relatively small island nation as a world superpower.

THE ORIGIN OF MODERN UNIVERSITIES

To successfully develop and pass on what we are calling "common understanding," universities must have certain immutable properties. One is that there must be a permanent faculty dedicated to the tradition of preserving knowledge. The preservation of knowledge is something that was picked up from the monastic system that developed in Europe after the fall of the Roman Empire in the fourth century. Between the fourth and eleventh centuries, that is for about 600 years, the political fragmentation of Europe, along with continuous external invasions from Arabs, Mongols, Tartars and others, made it almost impossible to sustain institutions of learning. Because of their religious connection, monasteries were relatively safer places for intellectual activity than other institutions during those turbulent centuries. The monasteries therefore became repositories of tradition, repositories in which libraries were maintained, scholarship valued, and knowledge preserved.

Things changed slowly during the eleventh and twelfth centuries when the European nation state began to develop. These larger aggregations of people were organized to meet external military threats. In addition, they also had the ability to concentrate resources and to open formerly closed intellectual explorations. Roger Bacon (1220–92) is perhaps the archetype of the kind of person who opened these new vistas and thereby created the modern university. It was Bacon's notion that the university should really have a function in addition to the preservation of existing knowledge, and that was the creation of new knowledge. It was Bacon who first provided the formula we still use in the search for new knowledge by laying the foundation of the experimental method.

Bacon taught that there was a portion of the discipline of philosophy that depended on believing what one sees and hears in the world and drawing experimental consequences from that belief. By developing this experience-based foundation for new knowledge, Bacon created a split in the classical discipline of philosophy and thereby ushered in what was then called "natural philosophy" or what we today call "science." This addition to the classic intellectual discipline of philosophy was the first of many fragmentations. It became the early seed from which increasingly specialized disciplines grew. Over the years, this expanding specialization has proved to be a mixed blessing. On the one hand, it has allowed scholars to find their way toward increasingly precise knowledge. On the other, a good argument can be made that when it comes to developing and passing on a common understanding of the world in which we live, many of the problems faced by universities today are a consequence of an overemphasis on specialized knowledge.

THE PARADOX OF SPECIALIZATION

At first, the creation of the discipline of natural philosophy did not change things substantially. New knowledge, or what today we would call the "frontiers of research," was an extremely small fraction of the university's life. However, during the fifteenth century, this began to change. The technology of navigation had progressed to the point where it became possible to conduct systematic explorations of the entire globe. A veritable explosion of knowledge resulted from these enterprises. In the process, enormous wealth was discovered elsewhere in the world and in many cases appropriated. People were quick to realize that to gain that wealth, it was necessary to have the technology and knowledge to conduct missions of explorations and conquest.

Henry of Portugal (1395–1460) is better known to history as "Henry the Navigator." It was he who realized that a small investment in the creation of new knowledge could yield enormous material rewards. It is no accident that Prince Henry established the first chair in mathematics, a subdiscipline of natural philosophy at the University of Lisbon. It is also no accident that ships sailing under Prince Henry's flag turned a small insignificant nation at the western tip of Europe into a major world power for over a century.

Efforts resulting from Prince Henry's support are perhaps the first graphic demonstration of the power inherent in the concerted application of new knowledge and technology. What happened during these years is that the well-known equivalence between knowledge and power became an article of faith with the monarchies emerging in western Europe. In the seventeenth century, this process became more formal, with the establishment of Royal Academies of Sciences in many European courts. In short, the search for new knowledge became a political imperative because it made successful conquests possible. This, in turn, made universities a resource that governments could not and did not ignore.

As the knowledge base expanded, so did specialization. By the nineteenth century, Roger Bacon's natural philosophy had evolved into physics, chemistry, mathematics, and the biological sciences. Today, of course, there are a multitude of subspecialities within each of these disciplines. It is now quite clear that this specialization is necessary if any progress is to be made in the creation of new knowledge. The clock simply cannot be turned back to the simpler time when it was possible for one person to be a walking encyclopedia. It is equally clear that this specialization has led to enormous increases in the wealth of society through the continued application of knowledge and to the wealth of the universities in which it is often created.

A good example of this is the story of what happened at the University of Marburg in Germany about a hundred years ago. In the final years of the nineteenth century, many research chemists in university environments spent their time synthesizing new compounds. Led by Emil Fischer, Fritz Haber, Gerard Willstatter, and others, German universities became the powerhouses of this particular form of high technology. Two professors of chemistry at the University of Marburg synthesized a substance called "acetylsalicylic acid" in 1877. One of them discovered quite by accident that the substance was a *mild analgesic* (in other words, a pain killer). The professor told this story to a friend who happened to own a textile mill in Marburg. It will not surprise too many readers that the name of the owner of that mill was Adolph Bayer and that acetylsalicylic acid is the substance commonly known as "aspirin." Aspirin was patented, and in 1900, commercial applications began. This process of university-based discoveries being transferred to the marketplace has been repeated over and over again, illustrating the importance of specialization and the advantage of specialization in the creation of knowledge and wealth.

Specialization cannot and should not be avoided. At the same time, it must be recognized that a price has been paid. This price is that the common understanding so central to the mission of the university has somehow been diluted. If the university consists solely of specialists and, more importantly, if the wealth of the university is created by some of these specialists and not by others, is it any wonder that other values of the university sometimes are ignored? It is the decline in the priority given to developing an inclusive perspective that now causes numerous problems for universities.

Again, an example is in order. In a 1989 proposal, *50 Hours: A Core Curriculum for College Students,* Lynne Cheney of the National Endowment for the Humanities (NEH) noted a midwestern university where students could choose from almost 900 courses ranging in content from foreign labor movements to the analysis of daytime soap operas. The result for students, at this and all too many other universities, is a curriculum constituted by, in the words of naturalist Loren Eiseley, "a meaningless mosaic of fragments." To better achieve a coherent "common understanding," the NEH has proposed what it calls a "core of learning." Whether we can all agree on what should be included in the core remains problematic. It is beyond dispute, however, that the specialized literature major who has no understanding of physics and the equally specialized engineer or chemistry major who graduates without studying history are both ill prepared to confront the complex choices they will face once they leave their universities.

SPECIALIZATION AND CONFLICT OF INTEREST

The fragmentation of knowledge inherent in specialization is only part of the problem. The link between specialized knowledge and the production of wealth presents an additional array of issues. About thirty years ago there was a professor at a major eastern university who was a consultant to a company manufacturing an automobile battery additive called "RDX-2." The professor analyzed the battery additive and made statements about the usefulness of the additive that the company used in its advertisements. Needless to say, the name of the university was prominently mentioned in the company's advertisements. In due course, the National Bureau of Standards got around to testing RDX-2, and the scientists there came to the opposite conclusion. They discovered that RDX-2 was essentially useless and subsequently published their results, as required by the bureau's charter. As one would expect, given that the corporation manufacturing RDX-2 had considerable political influence, a furor ensued. The corporation's influence was brought to bear, and the resignation of Allen V. Astin, then director of the Bureau of Standards, was forced. A number of congressional hearings followed, and finally Astin and his colleagues won their case, and after a year or so, he was reinstated.

This incident happened more than thirty years ago, but the problem has, if anything, become more common. In recent years, there have been charges of scientific and bureaucratic misconduct swirling around research on so-called cold fusion. In this case, a so-called discovery was announced in the press without the usual peer-review process required for publication in scientific journals. Similarly, allegations of questionable practices associated with cardiology research at Harvard University and research on drug treatments for retarded children with behavior problems conducted at the University of Pittsburgh have peppered the press in recent years. The list could go on and on.

Taken together, many of these allegations and questions involve what has come to be known as "technology transfer," wherein discoveries made in the laboratory are transferred to the wealth-enhancing arena of the marketplace. Such profit-making potential raises the possibility of a conflict of interest, which in turn may undermine the rigor of the scientific enterprise. It may also entail a *conflict of commitment,* where faculty members neglect their students and related academic duties to pursue lucrative products and research grants.

These issues are the subject of a controversial U.S. Congressional investigative report, "Are Scientific Misconduct and Conflicts of Interest Hazardous to Our Health?" released in September, 1990. This report, after providing the details of ten case studies, concluded that fraudulent practices had indeed been documented, that these practices had arisen in large measure from various conflicts of interest, that universities, including some of the most prestigious institutions in the country, had been reluctant to investigate the charges fully, that these same universities had acted in ways that encouraged retaliation against whistle-blowers, that the National Institutes of Health had ignored conflict-of-interest problems, and as a result, the public had been misled and endangered. In the process, the university's guiding mission—to reduce ignorance and to narrow the gap between knowledge and truth—had been perverted.

These are charges not to be taken lightly. Nor are the issues restricted to engineering and science. Financial and intellectual conflicts of interest in these fields have their counterparts in both the social sciences and the humanities. Lynne Cheney, chair of the NEH, lamented in 1988 that "viewing humanities texts as though they were primarily political documents is the most noticeable trend in academic study of the humanities today." Such a trend, Cheney went on to note, has made it easier to lose sight of the fact that the humanities "are about more than politics, about more than social power. What gives them their abiding worth are truths that pass beyond time and circumstance: truths that, transcending accidents of class, race, and gender, speak to us all."

What should universities do about this situation? Should they require all faculty to cut their ties with industry? Should professors refrain from involvement in the political arena? To what standards should members of a faculty be held? To what extent are universities responsible for investigating potential wrongdoings? All of these questions, as well as others, are common talk in the faculty clubs of our major institutions of higher education.

Requiring faculty members to sever their connections with the outside world would be a major mistake. There is no question that in fields such as engineering and business, such connections provide important reality checks and thereby very much enhance the educational process. Similarly, social scientists and scholars in the humanities who have firsthand knowledge of the ethical and empirical issues in such areas as biotechnology, civil rights, and the development of early childhood education programs are in a much stronger position to educate students than if they were required to retreat into disengaged scholarship in the halls of the academy.

In short, our students would suffer if we required our faculty to be totally isolated from the community. At the same time, incidents such as the one with RDX-2 must be avoided, and standards of behavior must be established that make it increasingly difficult for something like that to happen again. It is in the establishment of these standards that common sense and what we have called the "common understanding" come together.

THE COMMON UNDERSTANDING AND COMMON SENSE

First and foremost, there must be a strong affirmation of the principle that the preservation and pursuit of knowledge is the primary function of the university. As straightforward as this might sound, it must be restated because in recent years there has been a movement, popular in many quarters, insisting on the proposition that "feeling" is more important than "knowing." Thus, there are those who say that it is more important in a university setting to see to it that students "feel good" rather than that they "know more." Several pernicious consequences flow from this view, the worst being that the need to have universities at all goes away if this argument is carried to its logical conclusion.

Second is the point that of all the things that can be known, some are more important than others. It is here that the concepts of knowledge and of truth intersect. This is of critical importance because the difference between what might be called "trivial" knowledge and "serious" knowledge has to do with how what is known asymptotically approaches what we consider to be the "truth." Now, there are some who deny that there is such a thing as *truth*, arguing that the value of knowledge (its truth, so to speak) is all in the eyes of the beholder. This doctrine also is pernicious, in that it fundamentally undermines the purpose of the university. If truth is indeed only "in the eyes of the beholder," then why bother with education at all?

The questions raised in the preceding paragraphs have a direct bearing on the behavior of people in academic settings. If those who believe that truth does not exist and that all knowledge is relative prevail, then the search for truth becomes a charade, with the ultimate purpose of enhancing the influence of the searcher rather than expanding the horizon of human knowledge. Under such circumstances, it is much easier to succumb to the temptation to suppress experimental results that do not support a popular theory, or even to create research results, as we have seen in several well-publicized recent cases. It is also much easier to serve commercial purposes for financial gain if the very idea of truth is denied. With such a relativistic approach to scholarship, fraudulent or sloppy scientific research, as well as a humanities curriculum driven by a self-serving political agenda, may readily develop. What, after all, is the reason for a young graduate assistant or even an aspiring junior professor to worry about the truth of a research result or the value of a scholarly enterprise if there are distinguished senior professors on the campus who vehemently deny that there is such a thing as truth?

We who are members of the academy must continually guard against attacks on the very purpose of the institution. In general, when these attacks come from outside the university, they are relatively easy to counter. We close ranks and invoke academic freedom to win our point. When the attacks come from our own colleagues, however, they are harder to parry because they, too, will claim their privilege of "academic freedom." They will do this even as they deny the importance of knowledge or the existence of truth, thus undermining the foundations of the very institution they are supposed to serve.

Intellectual dishonesty in the academy has many facets. Those who seek to sell a political agenda under the guise of popular buzz-words such as "diversity" and "multiculturalism" are as guilty as those who manufacture research results to gain fame or fortune. Both are subverting scholarship for personal power or gain. Worst of all are the senior scholars who believe that they can do no wrong and that they must resist to the end all attempts by their academic peers and by the society at large to evaluate what they are doing. Academic freedom carries with it the heavy responsibility to behave in a way that maintains the public trust in academic institutions. In an environment where academic freedom is essential, this can only happen if the senior members of the academic community lead by the example of their own personal behavior.

Universities have served the human race well for almost a millennium. They have survived many crises before, and they will survive this one as well. By stressing the importance of knowledge and the pursuit of truth, and thereby working toward a common understanding of our civilization, the difficulties we have mentioned in this piece can be overcome. This is not only the beginning of wisdom; it is also simply common sense.

REFERENCES

Cheney, L. V. 1989. *50 Hours: A Core Curriculum for College Students*. Washington, D.C.: National Endowment for the Humanities.

U.S. House of Representatives. 1990. "Are Scientific Misconduct and Conflicts of Interest Hazardous to Our Health?" Nineteenth Report by the Committee on Government Operations. Washington, D.C.

5 • The Opportunities and Problems of Commercial Ventures: The University View

David A. Blake

To appreciate a university's rationale for establishing a for-profit subsidiary, one must first understand the reasons for academic interest in technology transfer. The term *technology transfer* is used to describe a bidirectional process through which the academic and commercial sectors exchange information, personnel, and new discoveries. The university undertakes efforts toward technology transfer primarily to enhance societal benefits from basic research and secondarily to capture a legitimate source of unrestricted income. Some believe that the profit motive is paramount in the academic sector. However, one has only to consider the relatively small size of this revenue source, even in the most successful universities, to realize its limitation. No university receives more than 5 percent of its research and development (R&D) support from technology transfer, and most receive less than 1 percent.

In recent years, municipalities have encouraged local research universities to use technology transfer approaches that result in the creation of new companies to stimulate local economic development.

It is important to appreciate that the formation of new corporate entities to accomplish technology transfer is but one of many approaches that are used. In order of increasing complexity, the modes of technology transfer are publication, research training (graduate students), faculty consulting, collaborative research, patent licensing, and creating a start-up company. Not only does the complexity increase along this list of modes, but also the cost to the investor and the potential for conflict of interest escalate.

Most discoveries from basic academic research do not lend themselves to immediate commercial exploitation. Because the creation of a new company represents a high risk to the investor, there is a built-in regulatory factor that dictates that the least expensive approach be used. Consequently, in the uncommon situation where a university invention can be marketed without further developmental research, patent licensing would be the expected route of transfer. However, most established companies are reluctant to utilize outside inventions, in part because they have their own R&D efforts, and R&D managers often see these as competitive. In the case of a seminal invention (e.g., a method of microbial genetic engineering), industry will immediately pursue the technology via patent licensing. In contrast, it is very difficult to license yet another monoclonal antibody-producing hybridoma, even if it can be shown to detect a cancer-associated antigen. Thus, the role of the start-up company is a legal vehicle for bringing together the discovery, the product champion, the venture capital, a management team, and the necessary facilities to develop a basic discovery to a point where commercial potential is more evident. The formation of a domestic start-up company also enhances American international competitiveness, whereas the licensing of inventions to foreign companies reduces competitiveness.

Universities are generally reluctant to become involved directly in the formation of a for-profit subsidiary or a spin-off company. There are many risks—all of them potentially damaging to the reputation of the institution in these ventures. Business failure is the number one risk. Most start-ups fail to develop the founding discovery into a commercial product or service. Business failure will disappoint the investors and the inventor. However, when the university only licenses patents to a company and does not take a direct role in that company, the academic institution is generally not held responsible for a business failure.

The other major category of risk is adverse publicity and resentment, particularly if the start-up company is successful. The public, through the media and the U.S. Congress, may question apparent university profits from successful commercialization of discoveries made during basic research funded through government grants and contracts. Established companies resent university start-ups because these start-ups are seen as draining off new technology the established companies view as competitive with their own business interests. Some corporate executives argue that universities are trying to get a bigger share in the profits. Even within universities, there may be resentment because faculty see university start-up companies as incompatible with the academic mission. It is argued that the allocation of resources and faculty promotions could be influenced by the prospect of institutional profit. All of these risks of adverse publicity stem from concern for conflict of interest. It does not really matter whether the conflicts are real or perceived because a university's most important asset is its credibility. Academic goals cannot be achieved unless the public, the media, government, industry, and faculty all have confidence in the university as a seeker and purveyor of truth. Derek Bok, president of Harvard University, said it well:

> With this bright promise, why does the prospect of technology transfer arouse anxiety on the campus of almost every research university? . . . For the great majority, however, the causes for concern lie elsewhere. They flow from an uneasy sense that programs to exploit technological development are likely to confuse the university's central commitment to the pursuit of knowledge and learning by introducing into the very heart of the academic enterprise a new and powerful motive—the search for commercial utility and financial gain. (Bok 1981)

Thus, the problem is one of balancing benefits and risks. It is self-evident that if faculty and universities have no stake in the commercial success of their research, there is no basis for the perception of conflict of interest. Is it realistic to expect faculty to be exempted from participation in the financial benefits of working in a capitalistic economic system? Will the best and the brightest basic scientists be willing to forego any financial reward for creative skills? Is it realistic to ask capital-starved universities to ignore a legitimate source of unrestricted revenues? Moreover, is it not a strategic mistake to minimize one of the most promising solutions to international competitiveness and balance-of-trade problems? The obvious answer is that we must find acceptable ways to effectively commercialize university discoveries, and that mission clearly requires dealing effectively with the conflict-of-interest issue. The problem then becomes defining an acceptable benefit-to-risk ratio and ensuring that the ratio is always maximized.

It is probably not possible to eliminate all perception of conflict of interest in technology transfer. The most benign mode of disseminating academic discovery is publication in the scientific literature, and yet there is escalating concern for bias among authors that have any ties with sponsoring companies. The lesson to be learned is that full disclosure is the first step in dealing with conflict of interest. Once the information is disclosed, the next step is to analyze the actual and possible conflicts of interest and to prescribe appropriate safeguards. In a sense, the start-up company is a means of managing conflict of interest. In a publicly traded company, federal securities regulations require the disclosure of all aspects of the company, including sources of technology, ownership, consultants, business risks, and so on.

However, what are the controls that could reasonably be expected to deal effectively with the potential conflicts of interest that arise when a university creates a for-profit company to commercialize university discoveries? There appear to be three major safeguards: (1) full disclosure, (2) an "arms-length" relationship between the university and the start-up, and (3) a nonexclusive relationship for both parties.

We have already discussed the need for full disclosure; it should be timely, complete, and public. An arms-length relationship means that the university does not control the governance of the company, nor does it dictate the company's business decisions. An arms-length relationship can be established through the formation of a *buffer organization* (i.e., an intermediate entity that provides a layer of insulation between the university and one or more technology-oriented start-ups). The buffer organization may be a not-for-profit foundation or a for-profit company. The university will probably appoint the majority of the board of directors of the buffer organization to ensure that it does not run away from its founding tie. The university generally retains some ownership in the buffer organization and thereby can share in the success of start-ups. An important advantage of a for-profit buffer organization is that it serves as a niche for professional technology transfer managers, many of whom thrive on compensation arrangements that are uncommon in academia.

The Johns Hopkins University has formed a buffer company—the Dome Corporation—which has a charter to develop real and intellectual property on behalf of the university and the Johns Hopkins Health System (hospital). Dome's Board of Directors is composed of Johns Hopkins trustees, corporate officers, and corporate leaders from the Baltimore community. Dome, in turn has formed another for-profit company—Triad Investors, Inc.—that is governed by an eight-member board, which is composed of five members appointed by Johns Hopkins and three appointed by the outside investors. None of the Johns Hopkins board members of Triad may be employees of Johns Hopkins. Thus, there are two layers of insulation between the university and the actual start-up companies that will be formed by Triad Investors. Triad will use its funds as seed venture capital, investing in promising new technologies emerging from Johns Hopkins or anywhere else. Triad is not obliged to work exclusively with Johns Hopkins, and the university has no obligation to give any favored treatment to Triad. The university employs technology-licensing specialists who work with faculty inventors and licensees. Triad will have no more or less access to these faculty inventors and university licensors than any other diligent prospective licensee. All of the usual institutional policies apply to arrangements with Triad. Triad has one edge, however—that is, it has a technology incubator building that is nearby the university and readily available for start-ups.

Triad is in its formative stages, and it is too early to assess its value and acceptance. It took two years to plan, largely because the university sought to satisfy all parties: trustees, deans, faculty, and potential investors. Even if Triad is successful as a seed venture fund, it is unlikely to change the research funding base of the institution. The Johns Hopkins University has a $400 million annual research budget (exclusive of its Applied Physics Laboratory) mostly from federal sources, and Triad's fund will not exceed $30 million, with an annual seed research investment of $3 million to $5 million.

Triad is not the first buffer organization created by a university to promote technology transfer. The oldest is WARF, which was formed by the University of Wisconsin as a foundation in 1925. The Massachusetts Institute of Technology (MIT) formed the MIT Development Foundation in 1972. More recently formed buffer organizations such as Dome/Triad have been for-profit companies. A partial list includes BCM Technologies, Inc. by the Baylor College of Medicine in 1984, Dallas Biomedical Corporation by the University of Texas at Dallas in 1986, and Medical Science Partners by Harvard Medical School in 1989.

The success of university spin-off companies should be judged on the basis of the companies' business successes and the absence of adverse effects on the mission of the academic institution. Management and minimization of inherent conflicts of interest is a key to the latter expectation. In the absence of an organization to create start-up companies, universities may be the unanticipated target of outside influences that seek to profit from university discoveries but have little or no regard for the reputation or integrity of the university. In this sense, one can see that a university buffer organization represents a positive step in the university's attempt to promote effective transfer of technology in an orderly fashion, while preserving a respect for academic values. The ideal formula for these buffer organizations is not yet known, but the quality of the academic institutions that have created them bodes well for a successful trial.

REFERENCE

Bok, D. 1981. Business and the academy. *Harvard Magazine*, 83: 26.

6 • Mechanisms of Interactions between Industry and the Academic Medical Center

Paul G. Waugaman and Roger J. Porter

The interactions between industry and the academic medical center are heterogeneous and complex. This chapter provides a framework for understanding these interactions through an analysis of the various essential elements involved in the interactions; ethical conflicts are dealt with in Chapters 7–10. First, we consider biomedical science's unique needs and approaches to scientific research. Next, the history of changing research patterns is considered, with emphasis on two dichotomous periods—before and after 1975. The most important concept follows, that of the five independent segments in academic-industry collaboration: (1) contract research, (2) consultantship, (3) employment, (4) technology transfer, and (5) gifts. All academic-industry interactions can be effectively analyzed by dividing the elements of each individual interaction—either potential or existing—into any or all of these segments.

Although research is an important activity for both industry and the academic medical center, the reasons why each undertakes scientific investigations differ greatly. For academia, research is partly an end in itself. The creation of new knowledge is a core mission of an educational institution—particularly a medical school. Sponsored research on the campus also provides the stimulus for a variety of other scholarly activities, such as the education of the next generation of scholars and the dissemination of new knowledge, both of which enhance the academic environment. Swept up in this research activity are the students, who are, ideally, exposed to the truth-seeking process, and the senior investigators, whose motivation is to better understand the nature of the biomedical world. Research is an integral part of the university.

For companies in the biomedical industries, research has a different role. Scientific investigation is a variably necessary part of the overall process of obtaining marketable products.

In the pharmaceutical industry, for example, many companies do no research at all, but merely market off-patent drugs at a lower price, or license others' technologies and concentrate on marketing and distribution. Research is most important for those large companies who can afford to be innovative in their approach to new therapies, and who expect to obtain not only a medical but also a financial return on the investment in research. The larger the company, the larger the research budget and the greater the expectation of eventual gains from new, patentable, innovative products. Research is also important to the small company organized to develop and exploit highly innovative new technologies or research tools. These firms usually lack production, marketing, and distribution skills. Instead, they concentrate on research and development. The emerging biotechnology companies of the 1980s exemplify this type of research-based company.

The differing roles of research in industry and academia translate into obvious differences in approach. In order to keep expenses to a minimum, businesses prefer to conduct and support research that is closest to application and marketing and directly relevant to the company's product line or target market. Such applied research, on the other hand, is less attractive to the traditional academician because it seldom adds to the fundamental understanding of nature in the way that more basic research will. Industrial research, therefore, is market driven, whereas academic research (in its purest form, at least) is knowledge driven.

Comparisons of engineering research to biomedical research are noteworthy, especially because academic-industry collaboration in engineering has a much longer history than in biomedical research. Most university engineering programs encourage faculty members to develop and maintain industry ties. In many engineering fields, professors are evaluated, in part, by their degree of industry involvement. However, engineering science is different from biomedical science. Engineering problems, by their very nature, tend to be applied and problem driven. Many research problems have practical applications in the near future; inventions are very often related directly to new products or to new manufacturing and processing methods. Fundamental science has a role in engineering research, but this role is relatively small compared to its role in biomedical research. Professors in the biomedical sciences have rarely been rewarded by their peers for their industry ties. The reasons for these historically weak ties are complex but are undoubtedly related in part to (1) the need for fundamental understanding of disease processes before any advances in therapy are possible, and (2) the readily available funds for basic biomedical research from the federal government.

Plentiful public support of biomedical science has created a group of basic scientists who are perceived by their peers and the public in general to be the most effective seekers of fundamental truths. Those who study applied biomedical problems have been considered less accomplished. Their work is considered ordinary and less prestigious. The best and the brightest in biomedical science have traditionally channeled their careers into basic research rather than the applied research that is more attractive to would-be industry collaborators.

Finally, biomedical research has one compelling difference from all other areas of science. Eventually, it involves humans who are tested with the new technologies or therapies. The application of biomedical science involves the highest social value—human life; therefore, such applications are subject to complex and costly reviews and regulation. The requirements for clinical trials of new drugs present a good example. Basic biomedical research or applied engineering research both enjoy the advantage of control of the experimental process, with more clearly defined outcomes. Basic biomedical research is usually cheaper and faster than clinical research. Applied biomedical research, including clinical research is—by comparison—expensive and slow, and it yields ambiguous results with surprising frequency.

These factors have all mitigated against applied biomedical research in general and academic-industry interactions in biomedical research in particular.

BIOMEDICAL RESEARCH AND ITS CHANGES, 1960–1990

Biomedical research has undergone many transitions, but the most important for the present discussion can be conveniently divided into approaches that antedate 1975 and those that have appeared since then.

Industrial Research before 1975

Before 1975, the biomedical industries emphasized clinical and developmental research. Basic research in industry was quite limited and was at the developmental end of the spectrum. In the pharmaceutical industry, for example, emphasis was on the screening of drugs for various biological activities rather than on the understanding of mechanisms of action involving such concepts as receptor sites. When fundamental research was undertaken by companies, it was to fill in the gaps in knowledge in order to facilitate development of new products or processes. Enthusiasm for basic research was low because of the long lead time from basic discovery to clinical applicability; industry funds for basic research were generally limited.

This is not to say that fundamental science was unimportant to industry. In general, however, the approach companies used was to collect the knowledge they required from other sources, typically from academia. Companies generally assumed that basic scientific information could be obtained without cost from the scientific literature and at scientific meetings. When necessary, literature and presented papers could be augmented through know-how obtained by hiring an expert professor as a consultant or hiring a recent graduate of the appropriate academic program.

Developmental research focused on problems such as formulation, production scale-up, and packaging. The emphasis was on product quality and on the reduction of costs in order to maximize the financial return of the marketed product.

Clinical trials, of course, have been necessary for much of this century, to obtain federal government approval for new products. The demand for even more extensive clinical trials of new drugs was increased dramatically by the 1961 Kefauver-Harris Amendment to the Food, Drug, and Cosmetic Act. This law also mandated that the efficacy of new drugs proposed for marketing be proven.

The industry has always assumed primary responsibility for the appropriate clinical trials for drugs or technologies that have a significant market potential. The pace of progress in the science of clinical trials has been driven by the requirements of government regulation, most notably by the U.S. Food and Drug Administration. Before 1975, the emphasis of pharmaceutical companies was on improving the methodologies for conducting controlled clinical trials, which at the time were relatively unsophisticated and, by today's standards, inexpensive.

Academic Research before 1975

Before 1975, fundamental biomedical research was marked by the long lead times from discovery to application to new products or processes. It was often difficult to draw direct relationships between the discoveries of cellular biology and the prevention and treatment of disease. The long lead times to application and the irrelevance of basic research to industrial problems generally limited industry's interest in fundamental biomedical research.

Because the opportunities to work on projects with potentially marketable products were limited, academic investigators tended to focus on the primary academic goal—knowledge accumulation—rather than on practical application or on the pecuniary rewards which might be associated with marketable products. In addition, fundamental research was adequately funded, primarily by the federal government but also by other sources such as foundations, further decreasing the need to seek out new players such as industry.

Before 1975, academic collaboration with industry in clinical research was better developed than in the basic sciences because of the need for clinical trials by industry. Academia is a natural source both for clinical expertise (the faculty), and for subjects for study (the patients). Before 1975, however, academic-industry collaborations were usually only at the end stage of the process; industry would first complete all the earlier studies, leaving only carefully defined, final studies for collaboration with academia. Academic investigators who became involved in such studies were often considered second-rate scientists who found it difficult to attain academic tenure; many physician-scientists became discouraged, turnover was high, and many followed the lure of private practice.

Industrial Research after 1975

After about 1975, the biomedical industry began to recognize that the lead time from discovery to market was shortening; an invention may have application in a much shorter time than was the case previously. Industry research began to take on some of the characteristics of academic research (Culliton 1982a).

In basic research, highly focused projects were now undertaken with the expectation that marketable products would eventually result. The process of mass screening of compounds began to yield to the new mechanism-oriented approach to diseases and their causes. Basic scientists who had been unexcited by the industry's screening approach to the search for new products found that the academic skills related to the understanding of disease mechanisms were greatly in demand; many became consultants to industry, and some chose to leave academia to work for companies. Others, encouraged by the potential applicability of their knowledge, formed companies themselves. The result has been the birth of new, research-oriented companies and a great expansion in the number and size of industrial laboratories doing fundamental research. An appreciation for this new biology, especially in biotechnology and molecular biology, has arisen in the corporate world.

Not only were basic inventions and processes viewed with a new value after 1975, but also some inventions coming from biomedical research clearly had multiple applications, even in areas distant from biomedicine itself (President's Biomedical Research Panel 1975). Lyophilization, for example, was developed through biomedical research—where its scientific importance remains undiminished—but the most important commercial application of lyophilization has been in the food-processing industry.

In clinical research, a new cost consciousness in industry became apparent. Clinical studies were more expensive and more closely supervised in order to protect investments and assure maintenance of schedules. Clinical study contracts were negotiated more carefully and expenses such as indirect costs were heavily scrutinized. A trend developed, for example, toward the use of contract (even mail-order) laboratories—instead of on-site university laboratories—to centralize and make more efficient the expensive process of patient testing and to obtain lower prices for some specific services. Market imperatives not only were thrust into the decision-making process but also became dominant over scientific research and scientific judgments.

Academic Research after 1975

In the years following 1975, basic scientists in academia, like those in industry, quickly recognized the shortening of the time from invention to application, and many began to reorient some of their priorities. Although interest in basic research remained unabated, interest in the applications of this research became a large factor in the minds of many. Scientists who were previously uninterested in the financial potential of their intellectual property—because, in general, it had little— were now thinking about ways to protect their knowledge and to benefit from it.

Not only scientists but also universities were quick to recognize the potential benefits of this newly valued intellectual property. Many universities formed internal units—in a variety of different ways—to protect their own interests in basic discoveries that occurred on their campuses. The impetus for pecuniary gain from this newly discovered potential source came not only from the natural desire of academic medical centers to maximize unrestricted income but also from the recognition that a gradual slowing in the rate of growth of federal support was inevitable—and that such slowing had already begun.

Clinical research after 1975 was confronted by several new variables. First, institutions became acutely conscious of cost recovery in expensive clinical trials and became more skillful in negotiating for all the costs of the research. On the other hand, the proliferation of outstanding academic clinical centers made the process more competitive; universities were now in competition with each other for clinical studies. In recognition of the need to be competitive, some academic centers formed "clinical trial centers" to enhance their posture and to suggest that added value was available when compared to the traditional approach of a single investigator dealing with a single company. Indeed, such centers have highly organized capabilities; the result is an improvement in the quality of important aspects of clinical studies, such as documentation, data collection, and patient follow-up.

Institutions have also become acutely aware of the legal aspects of conducting clinical studies. Academic medical centers now typically seek protection from the liabilities of clinical studies by carefully contracting with the company sponsoring the study. As liability insurance premiums climb, academic medical centers may begin to ask sponsoring companies to accept liability for all risks, including the negligence of their own investigators and staff. This will surely increase the degree of company direction and surveillance of clinical studies.

FEDERAL LEGISLATION AND ACADEMIC-INDUSTRY RELATIONSHIPS

Changes in federal law have also greatly altered the university's view of pecuniary gain from biomedical research. In 1980, the Bayh-Dole Act (Public Law [PL] 96-517) provided that inventions made by academic scientists on federally funded research projects were clearly subject to institutional policy and were not the property of the government. These incentives were reinforced by PL 98-629 in 1984. These laws have given universities the incentive to aggressively protect intellectual property and to seek industry partnerships to transfer technology into the marketplace. Also in 1980, the Stevenson-Wydler Act (PL 96-480) established a policy goal of speeding up the utilization of research results from federal laboratories. The Federal Technology Transfer Act of 1986 specifically gave federal agencies with in-house research laboratories, including both the National Institutes of Health (NIH) and the Department of Veterans Affairs (DVA), greater authority to protect intellectual property and to profit from the transfer of property rights to companies.

Universities are now encouraged to protect their intellectual property and to develop (often by license) the products that emerge from applied research. Collaboration with industry is a natural outgrowth of the self-interest that is stimulated by this legislation. The effect of the legislation has complemented the changes in the state of science as previously described.

From the standpoint of industry, the new laws provided new incentives for collaboration because corporations know more precisely what the university could actually negotiate. For the first time, industry could contract with the academic center and be certain that the university could indeed sell what it claimed to own. In effect, the academic medical center had obtained a form of title insurance for its intellectual property, even though this property was generated using federal funds.

This is not to say that all has been rosy in the collaboration with business. First, the benefits of these relationships have not been uniformly spread throughout academia. Companies have usually sought out scientists with the best reputations. Open competition is not the norm for industry-sponsored research. Consequently, industrial research tends to be concentrated in a few institutions. Second, companies are not uniform in their business dealings with universities, and practices differ from company to company, and often from project to project. University scientists and administrators are constantly off balance as relationships gel. This often creates misgivings about broadening or adding new collaborations. Third, business leaders continue to express disdain and impatience with universities' needs and points of view (Government-University-Industry Research Roundtable 1991). Finally, changes in tax law, corporate restructuring in an age of takeovers and acquisitions, and difficult market conditions all create instability in funding. This dismays academic scientists, whose activities usually move at a more leisurely pace. The consequent instability associated with industrial funds, especially in marginal situations, makes academic scientists wary.

CRITICAL ELEMENTS IN
ACADEMIC-INDUSTRY COLLABORATION

The management aspects of the relationships between academic medical centers and industry are as complex and heterogeneous as the scientific aspects of their common scientific problems. In spite of these complexities, however, the fundamental features of any relationship can be separated—surprisingly neatly—into five relatively independent elements. Any relationship between industry and academic medical centers can be analyzed by segmenting the features of the relationship into the following elements: (1) contract research, (2) consultantship, (3) employment, (4) technology transfer, and (5) gifts. Uncommon is the relationship that contains all five elements, but every relationship can be categorized into at least one of the five. Many relationships have features that fit at least two of the elements, with varying emphasis, depending on the needs of the partners.

The Contract Research Element

Contract research projects are, by far, the most common element in collaborative arrangements between industry and academic medical centers. Current estimates of the value of contract research sponsored by industry at universities approximate $350 million per year (National Science Foundation [NSF] estimates of national expenditures for research and development [R&D]). The fundamental tenet of contracted research is a specific request for particular research; the results are reported to the company (and usually somewhat later in scientific journals), and the company pays for the investigations. The results, obviously, may or may not be favorable to the company's plans for a product, but that is why the research is needed.

The research problem for a contract project is sometimes rigidly defined and may be the subject of extensive negotiation between the university (and its scientists) and the sponsoring company. The company may have considerable expertise regarding the problem and may wish to direct and review the academic work closely. A typical example might be a clinical trial, in which much of the design expertise, data collection, and statistical expertise, for example, resides in the company, while the knowledge of the specific disorder under study—and of course the patients to be studied—are the province of the university.

It is also possible to have a less rigid plan for research under the contract research element. The research question may be posed, for example, to a recognized expert with unique knowledge or unique techniques. This academic scientist may be given wide latitude to pursue the question asked, with little guidance regarding methodology. This approach is more typical of basic investigations and is often used to supplement the basic data developed in the company's own laboratories. The decision to use an academic laboratory is usually made on the basis of the need to have critical information about a product, combined with a relative lack of ability of the industry to perform the studies in-house without extensive retooling of their laboratories. In other words, a company believes it will be more cost-effective to perform basic studies by contract rather than in-house. With overhead costs rising in industrial research at the same rate that they are increasing in academia, and with more firms concentrating on the financial imperatives of the bottom line, this evaluation of the relative cost-effectiveness of contracted basic research will become more common.

The key document in this element is the *research agreement,* a contractual document setting forth terms and conditions for the relationship. Because there are more than 200 universities performing research sponsored by companies, and countless companies sponsoring academic research, models capturing consensus policies and practices have proven helpful. Two such compilations of models were published in the 1980s (Government-University-Industry Research Roundtable 1988; Society of Research Administrators 1984). Most universities have utilized these models, customizing them to reflect their unique policies, practices, or legal constraints. On the business side, most pharmaceutical companies have developed models for clinical trials, but not for basic research.

Intellectual property is often a result of contract research. The industrial sponsor will typically negotiate rights to this property as part of a separate technology transfer agreement, as described in the subsequent section on technology transfer element.

The Consultantship Element

Industry, in its own search for the best information about a potential or existing product, is continuously seeking advice from experts who may provide additional insight into both the positive and the negative aspects of the product. A consultation may be as simple as a phone call or it may be as complex as a standing commitment by an academic investigator to be available for several days per year to advise a company.

Consultantships, in themselves, are relatively straightforward transfers of knowledge from a faculty member directly to the employing firm. The gain to industry is clear. The gain to the university is indirect; consultants enhance the university's reputation by being chosen for their expertise, and the faculty members can supplement the university salary and be more content, presumably, without compromising obligations owed to the university as primary employer.

On occasion, consultants may have equity in the company for which they are consultants, or the consultants may receive stock as part of their compensation. In some cases, the consultant–faculty members may also be involved in a technology transfer from the university to the company, or even in contract research. Some universities limit the ability of the faculty member to play these multiple roles with the same company in order to avoid having conflicting interests.

The Employment Element

Companies often pay, in whole or in part, the salaries of university employees, especially entry-level scientists and graduate students. This may be handled through the university system, as research associateships or fellowships for graduate or postgraduate training. In some cases, company employees may work for specific periods in academic labs as guest workers. This arrangement may be mirrored by having academic faculty spend limited time in the company labs. Exchanges at this level are usually limited in time and purpose.

A frequent arrangement is that of a relatively informal process in which a university laboratory is supported by a company, with the expectation by both the laboratory chief and the company that the fellows and trainees who are company supported will be offered jobs by the company on completion of their training. Such arrangements usually depend on a strong personal relationship between the university scientists and their counterparts in the sponsoring company—that is, the company likes the people involved and the trainees that emerge. The benefit to the company is the availability of appropriately trained employees. For such an arrangement to succeed, the company must like the manner of education of trainees and must value their know-how acquired in the particular educational setting. The senior professor and the other permanent members of the university laboratory are often consultants to the company, usually by separate agreement.

Companies may also pay more senior members of a laboratory to work on specific projects by mutual agreement with the laboratory chief. Examination of potential conflicts of commitment and interest are important in such arrangements.

The Technology Transfer Element

Technology transfer concerns research that has proceeded to the point that invention has occurred, and it takes the form of licenses or start-up promotion. Over $80 million per year in royalties for invention licenses flow from companies to academic institutions (Atkinson and Forster 1991; Willey 1990). Royalties usually take one of two forms, either cash payments or stock in start-up or early-stage ventures.

The license agreement is the most common mechanism by which the university transfers technology to large companies. A patent or copyright is usually owned by the university, and the licensee company invests resources into the development, application, and marketing of the invention as a saleable product. The university collects royalties based on sales revenues, at a rate negotiated at the time the license is granted.

The start-up promotion is more heterogeneous and potentially complex. The invention is still owned by the university, but the company is typically a fledgling operation—often in need of venture capital. The company may be started by the inventor (usually a faculty member) or by an outsider, typically a local small business. The university may contract to perform some or most of the developmental experiments for the licensee—that is, the university may perform additional work on the invention, which is of an applied, developmental nature. The university collects royalties at a negotiated rate, usually without up-front payments, and often in stock rather than in cash.

Less commonly, and sometimes through a buffer company, the university may have a significant stake in both the research to transform an invention into a marketable product and the financial success of the product. The anxiety of universities becoming direct stakeholders in such ventures is considerable and is related to a number of complex considerations.

The Gifts Element

In its purest form, the gift is a transfer of resources without formal obligations. The gift transfer is from industry to an academic institution, is usually in the form of money, and involves neither the investigator nor the university being obligated to provide anything in return. A gift may be *conditional* (i.e., it may be "earmarked" for a specific research project, or a building, an endowed chair, the university endowment, or some other specific purpose). Most relevant to this discussion is a gift that is made to the laboratory of a specific university scientist.

The benefits to the university are primarily related to the lack of a formal obligation to provide anything in kind in return for the gift. Usually, there is no oversight by the donor company. The university runs a certain risk, however, that gifts are used by companies and encouraged by individual investigators to avoid paying indirect costs usually assessed on conventional research awards. If the gift is really an informal, paperless arrangement for the investigator to conduct specific research in a campus laboratory while avoiding payment of indirect costs, or overhead, to the university, the university may be the loser.

The benefits to the industry are several. The gift has tax advantages compared to a contract; also, if its intentions are truly philanthropic, it develops good relations between the institution and the company. On the other hand, a company may, if it trusts the investigator, avoid paying overhead to the university.

Gifts are often combined with other elements, including consultantships, employment arrangements, contracts, and/or technology transfer.

EXAMPLES OF ACADEMIC-BUSINESS RELATIONSHIPS

The variety and structure of academic-business relationships can be best understood using the foregoing five elements as one axis of an analytic matrix. The other axis of the matrix comprises an infinite variety of relationships. We suggest that the variety of relationships is infinite because the opportunity to make organizational innovations is limited only by the imagination and the creativity of the scientists and administrators involved in each relationship, the constraints of public law, and available money. None of these internal or environmental constraints have yet—in the authors' experience—limited the creation of new relationships. Although many relationships fall into a few categories because they have common characteristics, new variations constantly appear.

As academic-industry interaction—particularly in the biomedical sciences—has increased, relationships have tended to fall into some broad categories with common features. The following portion of this chapter analyzes three specific academic-business relationships in biomedical research and identifies and describes some other common relationships (Table 6.1).

This series of descriptions shows that a broad variety of relationships can be analyzed within the five distinct elements. It is not within the scope of this volume to provide more of the myriad possible examples.

The Product Development Relationship

The Becton Dickinson Corporation (B-D) sponsors research in the Infectious Diseases Section of the Department of Medicine at Wake Forest University's Bowman Gray School of Medicine. Robert Sherertz, an associate professor in the section, plans and organizes a program of laboratory and animal assays on the biologic action of polymers developed at B-D. B-D's commercial goal is the development of a line of bioactive devices that can be implanted in the human body for extended periods of time without eliciting the undesirable responses,

Table 6.1. Examples of the Elements Present in Academic-Industry Relationships

	Element				
Relationship	*Contract research*	*Consultantship*	*Employment*	*Technology transfer*	*Gift*
BGSM-BD Product Development	Yes	Yes	No	Yes	Yes
Georgetown University FIDIA Research Foundation	No	Yes	Yes	Yes	Yes
Washington University and Monsanto	Yes	Yes (Informal)	Yes (Informal)	Yes	No

Note: The elements are fixed, but they can be mixed as combinations representing the nearly unlimited number of possible relationships between industry and academia.

including immune and allergic reactions, anaerobic bacterial colonization, or blood clotting on the material surface.

The Contract Research Element

Sherertz has developed and described in publications unique methods for assessing biological activities in polymers in vitro and in animal models. B-D is interested in utilizing these assays to evaluate various polymer compositions at an early stage in their development, for their potential use in a broad variety of products. B-D's sponsorship includes support of Sherertz's research laboratory, including a technician, supplies, and materials.

The development of the polymers and the processes for including the biologically active substances in the polymer are proprietary to B-D. B-D therefore requires confidentiality on the part of Sherertz and his laboratory with this information. However, B-D has no objection to publication of results, so long as the company has the right to review publications to ensure that confidential information is not included. Sherertz has agreed to these restrictions and feels that the proprietary information will not be critical to the contribution to the literature made by publications he prepares.

Inventions or discoveries made by Sherertz's lab will belong to the school if they go beyond the composition of matter or potential uses claimed by B-D in patent applications or disclosures made before the evaluation of materials by Sherertz. However, B-D has the right to obtain exclusive rights through a royalty-bearing license, with such royalties to be negotiated at the time of licensing.

In addition to the laboratory studies, a second research agreement has been prepared to support clinical trials of devices, the initial activity of which is of sufficient interest to warrant studies in humans. These studies begin at the *Phase I level,* in that both efficacy and absence of adverse reaction is evaluated, again using controlled observations on volunteers with implanted devices. The clinical trials award is related to the cost of conducting individual experiments on volunteer human subjects, rather than on a time and effort basis, as are the basic studies. This second agreement provides for indemnification by B-D for any harm resulting from the use of their materials in accordance with the protocol in volunteer human subjects.

The Consultantship Element

Sherertz has a consultantship agreement with B-D that predates the establishment of the aforementioned research agreements. The agreement provides for Sherertz's advice and guidance to B-D with regard to the literature related to hospital infection or infections resulting from the implantation of reactive materials in the body. Sherertz also comments on published data for B-D and may review the company's confidential data and business plans in helping them choose polymers for further evaluation. Sherertz cannot do any original research work for the company under this agreement. Such original work will be done under the aforementioned research agreement. Sherertz is permitted to keep all consultant fees resulting from this relationship, and the consultantship agreement is subject to annual review and approval by his department chair and the dean of the medical school.

The Employment Element
None apply here.

The Technology Transfer Element
The laboratory research agreement was carefully negotiated with B-D to assure the company that it would have the initial right to review and obtain rights to any invention—whether patentable or not—made in the course of the research, as outlined in the scope of work. This would include any rights to patent applications where Sherertz or his colleagues at the school may be co-inventors with B-D employees. In the case of co-inventorship, the patent would be jointly held by the school and by B-D; and the school would be obliged to negotiate a license of its rights to the company for a fair royalty.

In the case of the agreement for the clinical trial, it is assumed that no inventions will be made, and that data will simply substantiate inventions made and claims filed in earlier stages of work. It is presumed, therefore, that B-D will either have licensed or hold total ownership of all proprietary rights.

This relationship has not resulted in any technology transfer arrangements.

The Gifts Element
This relationship began when Sherertz was a faculty member at another institution, and B-D's polymer business was in a smaller company. At that time, the company's business predecessor simply gave small amounts of money to Sherertz's institution to support his early research.

Subsequently, B-D acquired the business, and Sherertz moved to The Bowman Gray School of Medicine. As the size of the gifts became significant, B-D decided that it would be appropriate to cover the relationship with a formal agreement. At the same time, the medical school felt that it would also be appropriate to develop a formal agreement and to separate research to be done at the institution from Sherertz's responsibilities as a consultant to the company. It was at that time that it was mutually agreed to establish the foregoing research agreements.

The Enlightened Philanthropy Relationship

When a profit-making organization endows or supports a research effort without the common provisors such as prescription of research projects, access to inventions and other intellectual property, review of publications before public release, and the like, it can be termed *enlightened philanthropy*. The principal immediate commercial benefit for the sponsor is limited to publicity and goodwill. The rapid return through capturing and exploiting research advances is somewhat questionable.

In July, 1985, the representatives of Georgetown University and FIDIA Research Foundation (FIDIA R.F.), a nonprofit foundation supported by the Italian pharmaceutical company, FIDIA SpA, signed an agreement to create the FIDIA-Georgetown Institute for the Neurosciences. The institute is now housed in the facilities of the Georgetown Medical Center on the grounds of Georgetown University. In the near future, the institute will move to a new building at the university, which will be paid for by FIDIA R.F. The foundation also buys the institute's scientific and office equipment and pays for the institute's research expenses and the salaries of its sixty staff members. Georgetown University, for its part, brings to the venture its good name and the talents of its medical faculty.

The institute is legally not a separate corporate body but a division of FIDIA R.F. The institute is, in many ways, defined by its director. The director supervises the course of the institute's research and decides whether staff scientists can apply for research funds from external sources, such as National Institutes of Health (NIH). The director also makes final hiring decisions on staff members. Guidance of the institute's research directions is available from the institute's board of directors, which has the power to redirect the program, as necessary.

The Contract Research Element
None apply to this relationship.

The Consultantship Element
Scientific staff members may not consult with companies while employed at the institute. They are permitted, however, to perform routine academic exchanges of information and to give lectures at conferences and symposia. Scientists may even accept, with the director's

approval, honoraria to attend such gatherings, but this payment may not be viewed as payment for consultative services.

The Employment Element

The institute operates with a staff fluctuating in number between sixty and seventy people. Between forty and fifty people are nontenured, doctorate-level scientists, while up to ten are tenured Georgetown University faculty. The staff currently also includes eight support staff members. Staff members are employees of Georgetown University, but funds for salaries and benefits come from FIDIA R.F. Georgetown faculty members who are assigned to the institute cannot be assigned elsewhere without the agreement of the institute director, and, if assigned elsewhere, the university must assume responsibility for the faculty member's salary. Institute scientists recruited from outside the university are recommended for Georgetown University faculty status, as appropriate, and all institute staff have all the rights and privileges of comparable Georgetown University employees.

Institute scientists perform their research under supervision of the director. In addition, they may teach and take part in other scholastic activities at Georgetown University for as much as 30 percent of their time.

The Technology Transfer Element

FIDIA R.F. has first rights to patent any invention developed through research at the institute, but there is no agreement that any particular organization will be awarded licenses to utilize institute patents. There are seven directors on the board, and FIDIA R.F. can influence licensing decisions through their four representatives on the foundation's board of directors. However, final approval of license awards requires a majority of five votes. If FIDIA SpA receives a nonexclusive license, it is required to pay royalties no less than any other licensee. Although the policy of Georgetown University provides for sharing royalties received with inventors, all royalties from institute inventions are retained by the institute.

The Gifts Element

The new building for the institute on the Georgetown campus is effectively a gift to the university. The only condition is that the institute be permitted to occupy the building until the bonds sold to finance the building are paid off. The university will issue the bonds and will supervise construction. FIDIA R.F. will include payment of principal and interest due in its grant to the university to operate the institute.

The Strategic Alliance Relationship

The strategic alliance relationship has emerged in the 1980s as a long-standing relationship involving a single company and a single academic institution. The term generally defines a situation where a company will support a number of projects within an institution simultaneously. The alliance is marked by an important strategic decision by the company to make a major, multiyear commitment to support a research effort that may not have a direct and immediate benefit to the company's businesses or product line, but that may signify a long-term investment in improved know-how and advanced state of the art for the company. An important element of that decision is to concentrate the investment in a single institution or laboratory, for whatever reason.

In July, 1982, the Monsanto Corporation and Washington University in St. Louis initiated a strategic alliance in the field of biomedicine, with a focus on "proteins, peptides, and other molecules which modulate cellular function" (Culliton 1982b). The initial agreement was for a five-year period through 1987. The agreement provided for a gradual buildup of support to the level of $5 million per year in 1982 dollars. In 1985, support was adjusted upward for the final two years, so that the total value of the first five-year period was more than $30 million. The agreement was extended in 1986 and 1990 and is currently scheduled to continue through 1994. The practice of increasing the annual award based on the gross national product inflation index has raised its annual value to approximately $9.2 million. Anticipating adverse business conditions in 1990, 1991, and 1992, the parties agreed to forgo the increase for inflation in those years. Indexed increases will resume in 1993 and 1994.

The technical scope of the alliance and the general principles of operation were established jointly by David Kipnis, professor and chair of the department of medicine at Washington University, and the late Howard Schneiderman, vice president for research at Monsanto at the time. Schneiderman had been dean of the School of Medicine at the University of California at Irvine before joining Monsanto in the early 1980s. As the agreement was being structured, several scientists from both the Washington University faculty and the Monsanto staff participated in the discussions.

The Contract Research Element

The contract research element is the most visible and formal part of this relationship. Each year, Washington University faculty members may propose research projects for inclusion in the overall research program. Projects are selected for funding by a ten-person steering committee chaired by Kipnis. Five members of the steering committee come from the faculty of the university, and five from Monsanto. The steering committee evaluates scientific merit and ranks the projects for funding. Prior to soliciting proposals each year, the steering committee provides the faculty with a statement of funding goals and objectives, as part of the call for proposals. Officials of both the university and the company claim that the company does not exert undue influence in this process. The overall agreement stipulates that the research in the program will be approximately 30 percent basic and 70 percent applied. However, this ratio is not considered by the steering committee at the time projects are selected for support. Company officials, however, indicate that the mix is reviewed after support decisions have been made, and adjustments would then be made in the next year's call for proposals (MacCordy 1991).

Projects may be funded for up to three years. However, the steering committee may approve projects for a shorter period of time if they feel that work cannot proceed for three years without some review.

The steering committee may also adjust project budgets on the basis of scientific review. For example, equipment may be deleted from a project's budget if the steering committee members know that other equipment may be available on a shared basis, or if they believe that equipment will be superfluous to the research proposed. The university's indirect costs are also included in the project budgets. Indirect costs are pegged at a rate negotiated for the entire award period. University officials indicate that this rate has not changed since 1982, although opportunities have existed to adjust the rate at each of the two renewal negotiations (MacCordy 1991). The university agreed, however, that the rate would remain constant for each renewal period.

The Consultantship Element

Several Washington University faculty members who have been engaged in the program since 1982 have served as consultants to Monsanto. Such consultantship arrangements are not formally linked to the agreement or other aspects of the arrangement but generally stem from the close geographic proximity of Washington University to Monsanto and the close scientific relationship between Monsanto's principal research activities in the St. Louis area (synthetic chemistry, plant biology, and biotechnology) and the scientific expertise of Washington University faculty members. Consultant relationships are governed by Washington University's existing policies for review and approval of such outside activities (which may be for limited commitments of time in the case of the medical school faculty).

There is no specific prohibition of faculty members working on projects included in the arrangement otherwise serving as consultants to Monsanto simultaneously. Both the university and the company would take pains in such a case to ensure that conflicts of interest would be avoided. Consultantship arrangements are subject to annual review and approval by a faculty member's department chair.

The Employment Element

As with the Consultantship, there is no formal portion of the arrangement that establishes a personnel exchange between the university and the company. However geographic proximity and common interests often result in mobility between Monsanto staff and university faculty. Presently, two former Washington University faculty members now serve as key science executives at Monsanto.

Initial plans for the arrangement anticipated a major influx of Monsanto scientists into Washington University labs to be full-time collaborators in research projects (Culliton 1982a). This has not materialized to the extent expected, largely because the scientists within Monsanto have higher priorities.

Graduate students who catch the eyes of Monsanto monitors and who want to stay in the St. Louis area are naturally likely to get job offers. Neither the university nor the company have formally tracked the hiring of graduate students because this is not a formal element of the arrangement.

The Technology Transfer Element

The agreement specifies that Monsanto will have an opportunity to review publications or presentations resulting from projects included in the program. This review allows Monsanto to file any patent applications necessary to protect patent rights.

Monsanto also has the right to obtain exclusive licenses to any patents resulting from research. The agreement clearly limits Monsanto to patents only, and not to know-how. Scientists participating in the project generally disclose directly to Monsanto (through the project monitor assigned by Monsanto). Monsanto then takes responsibility for preparing and filing patent applications in the university's name.

Monsanto's goal is to develop a market-oriented patent position relative to a technology of interest. The company believes that an important strategy for attaining that objective is to assume that patents of particular interest to it will be filed and pursued. The university also believed that it did not have the staffing or financial resources to pursue these matters and that Monsanto was in a better position to do so. The strength of the commercial patent position is a key element in the value of the arrangement to the company. Officials of the university and the company believe that the practice has meant that far more patents have been applied for and obtained because of this interest than would have otherwise been the case.

If Monsanto is not interested in pursuing an invention, the university is free to do so at its own initiative or to return the rights to the faculty member. The return of patent rights is a rare occurrence.

When the arrangement began, Schneiderman (of Monsanto) was optimistic about the potential to create new products and processes for Monsanto. "If everything works right," he said, "we'll see a few products approaching the marketplace by the end of the decade, given luck and a few people lighting some candles" (Culliton 1982a). Apparently, the right candles were not lit. S. Allen Heninger, a vice-president of Monsanto and president-elect of the American Chemical Society, reported that the arrangement cannot be judged yet, but to date, no products have been developed. Furthermore, he said that "at this point in a well-run in-house project, Monsanto would have expected products by now" (Government-University-Industry Research Roundtable 1991).

The Gifts Element
None apply to this relationship.

Other Relationships

The following brief descriptions address some of the common academic-business relationships beyond those covered in the preceding three examples. They are presented in summary descriptive form without reference to specific examples.

The Multisponsor Consortium
In this situation, a number of companies that may be competitors, but that have common scientific interests and research needs, will contribute jointly to an academic research program. Generally, the research program is composed of two or more discrete research projects and two or more scientists. Research priorities are established collaboratively, with each sponsor having equal voice in decisions. Research results from the program are available to all industry participants, usually before general publication. Inventions are available to all spon-

sors. Sometimes, royalties are forgone. Individual companies may also sponsor proprietary or other targeted research without sharing results or information with the other participating companies.

The prototype for these consortia are generally found in the University/Industry Cooperative Research Centers Program of the NSF. The NSF has provided start-up and developmental support for fifty-seven such centers since 1979. Currently, forty-five centers are operational (Schwartzkopf 1991). Each center has several member companies supporting its research program. Most of these centers address problems of manufacturing technology and other technologies outside the biomedical field. One center, the Center for Cell Regulation at the University of Texas Health Science Center at San Antonio, is related to biomedical science, and two other centers are concerned with aspects of biotechnology.

The Faculty Start-up

In this relationship, a faculty member with sufficient interest in commercially developing a research advance will organize a company. This commercial venture may have the backup (both financial and managerial) of a qualified entrepreneur or of a venture capital syndicate, or it may be solely supported by the faculty member and members of her or his immediate family or close friends.

In many of these relationships, the inventor/scientist's academic institution will support the venture in nonfinancial ways, such as providing release time to pursue commercial interests, rental of research laboratory space or access to special research resources at favorable rates, and access at favorable terms to intellectual property rights held by the university. These relationships permit an inventor/scientist to retain a working participation in development efforts that may not be an appropriate academic endeavor, or that may be impossible in academic laboratories because of space limitations or the need for maintaining trade secrets or other commercial proprietary considerations.

Faculty start-up ventures are usually quite dynamic and can be expected to go in one of three directions: (1) Probably the most common scenario is one in which the venture limps along at a low level of effort for a number of years, fails to fulfill the scientific goals and objectives, and falls apart when available capital is expended. (2) The venture proceeds satisfactorily through the proof-of-concept commercial aspects of the research advance to the point where an established company with the financial resources to market the technology buys out the start-up venture, to the considerable financial benefit of the entrepreneurs and their financial backers. (3) The company grows and moves from a research stage to a manufacturing and marketing stage. In this case, it is usually necessary for the faculty members who started the company to choose between the company and their faculty responsibilities. If they choose to stay with the company, the faculty members become businesspersons. If they choose to remain primarily academics, they are usually forced into the position of giving up control of the management of the company and to become nonparticipatory directors or, in some cases, the beneficiaries of a buy-out.

The Third-Party Start-up

This relationship may be almost the same as the faculty start-up. However, the critical difference is that the impetus to establish a venture around an academic research advance or a cluster of advances comes from an outside party. The outside entrepreneur, often with the support and cooperation of the academic institution's administration, encounters a promising academic research advance, assesses the commercial potential of that advance, assembles the necessary capital to pursue the commercialization effort, and provides management leadership and direction to the effort.

In many instances, the inventors/scientists may commit themselves to work with the new venture, perhaps as research contractors or consultants, and the institution collaborates with the entrepreneur through a license arrangement or through some other mechanism for maintaining academic sanction of the relationship. The outcomes of these relationships usually follow the same three alternative directions as the faculty start-up. However, the inventors/scientists usually do not become as involved or commit as much of their time with regard to the commercialization effort as the inventors/scientists who are engaged in managing their own start-up venture.

Summary

Each of the preceding examples is relatively common. There are several variations on these general types, and additional types could be described and elaborated if space permitted. However, it is evident from these examples that the segments of any type of relationship can be readily understood in the context of a relatively few and easily differentiated descriptive segments, which can characterize the full extent of any type of relationship.

The preceding examples demonstrate that even given the complexity and variety of biomedical academic-industry research relationships, these relationships can be analyzed and compared by reducing them to a manageable series of common elements, then comparing their characteristics to those in other situations. In this way, it may become easier in the coming years to evaluate objectively the effectiveness of the approaches for each element and to improve overall models.

REFERENCES

Atkinson, S. D. and Forster, M. "Survey of Academic Technology Transfer." Presentation at Association of University Technology Managers Annual Meeting, San Francisco, February 25, 1991.
Culliton, B. J. 1982a. The academic–industrial complex. *Science,* 216: 960.
Culliton, B. J. 1982b. Monsanto gives Washington U. $23.5 million. *Science,* 216: 1296.
Government-University-Industry Research Roundtable, National Academy of Sciences, 1988. *Simplified and Standardized Model Agreements for University-Industry Cooperative Research.* Washington, D.C.: National Academy of Sciences.
Government-University-Industry Research Roundtable, National Academy of Sciences, 1991. *Industrial Perspectives on Innovation and Interaction with Universities.* Washington, D.C.: National Academy of Sciences.
MacCordy, E. L. and Williams, J. W. Personal interview. March, 1991.
National Science Foundation. 1991. *Estimates of National Research and Development Expenditures, 1991.* Washington, D.C.: National Science Foundation.
President's Biomedical Research Panel. 1975. *Report on the Application of Biomedical Research.* Washington, D.C.: U.S. Department of Health, Education, and Welfare.
Schwartzkopf, A. J. Personal interview. January, 1991.
Society of Research Administrators. 1984. *Guide to University-Industry Research Agreements.* Santa Monica, California: Society of Research Administrators.
Willey, T. 1990. *A Study of Selected University Technology Licensing and Technology Transfer Programs.* Indianapolis: Indiana Corporation for Science and Technology.

OTHER READINGS

Blumenthal, D., Gluck, M., Louis, K. S., et al. 1986. University-industry research relationships in biotechnology: Implications for the university. *Science,* 232: 1361–66.
Blumenthal, D., Epstein, S., Maxwell, J. 1986. Commercializing university research. *New England Journal of Medicine,* 314: 1621–26.
Culliton, B. 1982. The academic-industrial complex. *Science,* 216: 960–2.
Culliton, B. 1990. Monsanto renews ties of Washington University. *Science,* 248: 1027.

Marshall, E. 1990. When commerce and academe collide." *Science,* 248: 152–6.

The payoff in funding university research. 1986. *Business Week,* 2593: 76.

Government-University-Industry Research Roundtable, National Academy of Sciences, 1989. *Science and Technology in the Academic Enterprise—A Discussion Paper.* Washington, D.C.: National Academy of Sciences.

PART III

The University Medical Center's Inward View of Collaboration with Industry

7 • Conflicts of Interest in Research: The Fundamentals

Roger J. Porter

HISTORICAL PERSPECTIVE

In the search for historical verities that may contribute to our current understanding of conflicts of interest in research, we must first consider that most fundamental of all human investigative characteristics, the power of observation. Observation, after all, is the beginning of empirical science, and although the more sophisticated deductive process is usually emphasized when considering conflict of interest in research (as in Chapter 9, for example), the scientific process starts with our vision of nature. An adequate consideration of human observational capabilities should first consider our limited ability to observe properly, followed by an analysis of how to improve observational power by manipulation of the environment. The first might be called the "limitations of observational truth" and the second, the "enrichment of observational truth." Clearly, a very broad definition of observation is used here.

The Limitations of Observational Truth

The limited nature of human powers of observation has been discussed since the earliest Greek writings. Although Plato was uniformly skeptical about the real nature of objects, he especially noted the interference by the body on objective observation, noting that "the body disturbs . . . and hinders the soul from getting possession of the truth" (Rouse 1956). Plato expanded by noting that "if we do have some leisure, and turn away from the body to speculate on something, in our searches it is everywhere interfering, it causes confusion and disturbance, and dazzles us so that it will not let us see the truth." Further, "it is impossible in company with the body to know anything purely" (Rouse 1956). Aristotle carried the concept further, by noting that "we have the power to imagine things whenever we please, seeing them in our mind's eye" (Wheelwright 1951).

We have not been able to improve on the skeptical views of these ancient Greeks. Subsequent data, in fact, have increasingly supported their pessimistic view of the powers of human observation. Humans are plagued by this inability to observe "purely," although science has altered our approach to data acquired by observation. It is inherent in the nature of science that observation is held to a very high standard of preestablished impersonal criteria—the objectivity that forms the characteristic of "universalism" described by Robert Merton: "Scientific claims are not to depend on the personal or social attributes of their protagonist; [their] race, nationality, religion, class, and personal qualities are as such irrelevant." Objectivity derives from the "impersonal character of science" (Merton 1973).

Do our observational powers really fail us, though? Are we really so weak in this modern, enlightened era that we cannot discern truth from falsehood? A recent example from biomedical research is appropriate:

> Based on certain anecdotal data and preliminary studies, as well as on a highly logical and sound expectation from fundamental scientific knowledge, the drug encainide was marketed for use in patients with ventricular arrhythmia, a potentially life-threatening abnormality of cardiac rhythm. The drug was relatively well accepted and was marketed by a highly ethical pharmaceutical company. Its safety was also accepted, and, in the 1989 *Physicians' Desk Reference* (p. 717), the drug was noted to be "effective in treating ventricular arrhythmias in patients with and without organic heart disease." The critical observations appear to be complete.
>
> However, because previous studies had emphasized the issue of arrhythmia suppression rather than clinical outcome and because of other uncertainties regarding encainide (and a sister compound flecainide), the drug was subjected to a multicenter, randomized, placebo-controlled study to see whether the drug reduced the death rate in asymptomatic or mildly symptomatic patients. Encainide and flecainide, after an average of ten months of follow-up, caused more deaths than placebo (Cast, 1989), by a factor of more than two to one. What had appeared to be sound observation was, on careful examination by a rigorous study, not true. Clearly, the intuition of many physicians was incorrect (Passamani 1991,

p. 1591). The 1991 *Physicians' Desk Reference* now states that encainide is "indicated for the treatment of documented ventricular arrhythmias," and "should not be used in patients with less severe ventricular arrhythmias, even if the patients are symptomatic" (p. 700). Lives will be saved by the resulting improvement in our understanding of this drug.

The search for better means of observation is the continuous and unrelenting effort of science. In clinical trials, for example, "rather than continue to choose among therapies whose relative benefits are in dispute, a physician initiating a randomized clinical trial makes the intellectually honest admission that best therapy is not known, and that an ethical course of action is to undertake a randomized clinical trial to find out" (Byar 1976).

Sometimes, the scientific observations appear to be quite intact, but emotions prevent the acceptance of the data. The following example shows how objectivity can be blurred even in the face of impeccable observation.

In a randomized, double-blind cross-over study of a new drug for epilepsy, patients with uncontrolled seizures were told that they could continue on the new medication at the end of their participation in the study, only if their seizure frequency had been decreased by the addition of the new drug. Because each patient was on placebo during part of the study, and because neither the patient nor the physician-investigator knew when the patient was taking the new drug or the placebo, seizure counts were completely objective. All patients agreed in advance that if improvement did not occur while taking the new drug, the patients would be discharged on their former, admittedly inadequate, standard medications.

As might be anticipated by those with some experience in clinical trials, the moment of truth came as a tremendous relief to those who were helped by the drug, and an unfathomable blow to those who were not. What was remarkable, however, was the discovery that *all* patients wished to continue on the new drug, even those for whom the drug was documented to be ineffective! The hope for a new, more effective medication completely overwhelmed the objective observations provided to the patient by the study.

These examples show how observations may prove to be false, even when seemingly well grounded, and how objective interpretation of good observations may be influenced by less-than-objective, emotional factors. These examples also document one of the most important scientific challenges in modern medicine, that of discerning whether a medication is or is not effective. However, would physicians in an uncontrolled study have been more objective on behalf of their patients? Are their observational powers superior? This issue is fully addressed in Chapter 9, but fundamentally, the answer is "no." As noted by Northrup (1983), "the natural scientist . . . , in his immediately apprehended data, is confronted with factors which are personal and private and relative."

The Enrichment of Observational Truth

If our observational powers are so innately dismal, what might we do to enhance these powers and come closer to the truth? The answer lies in a manipulation of the process, an *experiment,* which enhances the objectivity of our observations. As noted by Meinert (1986), the use of experiments—even with humans—is not at all new. The Book of Daniel (Daniel 1:12–15) describes a planned clinical study lasting ten days and utilizing two groups, one tested against the other. So even the earliest observers anticipated their own frailties and designed experiments to overcome their observational limitations. Other examples, as noted by Pocock and Meinert, include observations by Pare on the treatment of battlefield injuries in the sixteenth century and the experiments of Lind in determining the curative powers of citrus fruit on scurvy in the eighteenth century.

Progress has been slow, however. It was fifty years after Lind's observations that the British Navy first provided lemon juice to its sailors (Pocock 1983), and not until the nineteenth century that Louis— using multiple observational groups—found bloodletting to be an ineffective therapy. The scientific basis of clinical trials and epidemiology has only slowly become accepted; it was not until the second half of the nineteenth century that placebo-controlled studies were advocated and the early twentieth century that randomization was recommended (Meinert 1986). Each of these refinements enhances the objectivity of the observational powers of the investigator. Skepticism of one's observational powers is the first line of defense in the fight for objectivity (Merton 1973), and the experiment is the conversion of this skepticism into an organized truth-seeking effort. Randomization and blinding are embellishments on the experiment, designed to prevent external influences such as conflict of interest from tampering with this objectivity.

In addition to the slow pace of making even elementary use of scientific approaches to attack difficult problems, similar tardiness has been associated with the recognition of key factors that damage objectivity. A relatively recent example is found in one of the most influential of academic conflict of interest documents, "On Preventing Conflicts of Interest in Government-Sponsored Research at Universities," published in 1964 by the American Council on Education (Council of the American Association of University Professors and the Council on Education 1964). This document, which is less than three decades old, does not even mention bias in research! It admonishes both the government and institutions of higher learning to set standards for conflict of interest but describes only administrative issues (see the following section). This failure to address bias in research is surprising, especially considering that concepts of randomization and the need for bias control had been emphasized for many years. I am reminded (Jonas Ellenberg, personal communication, February 1991) that the academic community waxes and wanes in its enthusiasm for compulsive bias control in research, and that even in the 1980s, attempts have been made to circumvent controlled trials with less rigorous evaluations. Fortunately, the trend toward scrupulous bias control remains clear (Porter 1990).

CONCEPTS AND DEFINITIONS

Although the argument is often made that conflicts of interest are not inherently bad (Bray 1990), the very nature of a conflict suggests that a problem exists. Conflicts of interest have been variously defined, but the best summary is the oldest: "No one can serve two masters, for either he will hate the one and love the other, or he will be devoted to one and despise the other. You cannot serve God and mammon" (Matthew 6:24). A person with a conflict of interest has two masters to serve, and these two masters do not always have coincident needs. Conflict of interest can never be, in its entirety, a good event, as one of the masters usually must lose.

It is certainly true, of course, that identifying a specific conflict of interest is difficult. As one respected reporter noted, "conflict of interest, like pornography, tends to defy simple definition: one researcher's conflict of interest is another's mutually beneficial working relationship" (Palca 1989). It is also an oversimplification to say that scientific motivations are *always* in conflict when two masters are served. When the two masters appear to have coincident interests, then the conflict may be best described as a *potential* conflict of interest.* Theoretically, at least, the two masters must have divergent interests in the same endeavor for conflict to be present. Unfortunately, the boundaries of

---

*I am not using the term *potential conflict of interest* in the sense of an event that has yet to occur (i.e., anticipation of conflict of interest); *potential conflict of interest* is used here when two masters already exist, but no obvious conflict is yet apparent.

what is a potential conflict of interest and what is a genuine conflict of interest are fuzzy and in the eye of the beholder. Investigators who wish to downplay conflict of interest in their research often refer to the serving of two masters as a "potential" problem, whereas others—perhaps more objectively—may simply call it "conflict of interest." Nor should all conflicts of interest be avoided. For example, the role of a talented consultant—who may also have equity in the company—in bringing a product to the marketplace may be invaluable; such a person may play a very positive, constructive role (Sabean 1989).

In research, conflicts of interest can be at either the individual or the institutional level; the latter is addressed in Chapter 4. For an individual, the conflict is usually one in which the truth-seeking scientific endeavor has been unwittingly subverted for other gains—usually fame or fortune or both (see Chapter 8). The following are concepts that require further definition and discussion.

Administrative Conflicts

The vast majority of conflicts encountered in the university (indeed in any organization) have little to do with the influence of conflict of interest on research results and interpretation. Instead, most conflicts are what one might interpret as "administrative," concerned with matters such as favoring outside interests in business dealings with the university, undertaking research (or other activities) without informing the university, purchasing equipment for university research from a private company in which the faculty member has a financial interest, inappropriate transmission of data for personal gain, influencing of contracts for personal gain, and so on (Council of the American Association of University Professors and the American Council on Education 1964). None of these directly involve the focus of the impact of conflict of interest on research, which is to produce biased results or biased interpretation of results, and which is the focus of the chapters in this volume.

The Appearance of Conflicts

The *appearance* of conflicts of interest is, of course, the public perception independent of the facts. The appearance of conflicts of interest may be related to (1) genuine conflicts of interest, (2) potential conflicts of interest, or (3) the genuine absence of conflicts of interest despite appearances to the contrary. It is public perception, however, that fuels the engine of regulation; such perception is therefore of the

utmost importance—not so much for determining the truth but for controlling the impact of public opinion and governmental intervention.
Government employees are under especially strict guidelines to avoid conflict of interest in their activities, both official and unofficial. The perception is as important as the activity: "The activity itself, standing alone, may be acceptable, but the involvement with the other party may not. The intent of the employee may be innocent, but that is immaterial. It is the perception of the critical taxpayer that counts" (Rasinski 1987). The issue is also relevant to the private sector, however, as noted by the Councils on Scientific Affairs and Ethical and Judicial Affairs of the American Medical Association: "Even the mere appearance of a conflict of interest may be sufficient to denigrate a research project, investigator, university, or corporation" (Council Report 1990).

Self-deception and the Unavoidability of Conflicts

Although conflicts of interest are never good, many are unavoidable. Investigators constantly make decisions that can influence the results of an experiment; the motivations for these decisions are an inextricable mixture of the search for truth, fame, and fortune. Decisions must be made, and as no yardstick yet exists for measuring their purity, many are undoubtedly influenced by factors other than the search for truth. Some investigators disagree with this rather downbeat assessment of scientific candor. I have found useful the following summary of conflicts of interests, which describes the difficulty that physicians face when accepting favors from a drug company; this is not conflict of interest in research, but the principle is the same—just substitute "scientist" for "doctor":

> Few doctors accept that they themselves have been corrupted. Most doctors believe that they are quite untouched by the seductive ways of the industry's marketing men; that they are uninfluenced by the promotional propaganda they receive; that they can enjoy a company's "generosity" in the form of gifts and hospitality without prescribing its products. The degree to which the profession, mainly composed of honorable and decent people, can practice such self-deceit is quite extraordinary. No drug company gives away its shareholders' money in an act of disinterested generosity. (Rawlins 1984)

I respectfully submit that such "self-deceit" can also be practiced by scientists who serve two masters, even though scientists are also mainly honorable and decent people.

On the other hand, in defense of physicians' discriminatory powers, the pharmaceutical industry mounts a strong rebuttal: "It is demeaning to the profession to suggest that doctors are unable to disregard information in which they have no interest; doctors must be critical and can accept or reject what they will" (Wells 1987). Furthermore, a 1991 survey of 3000 physicians suggested that most physicians do not think that honoraria affect their clinical judgment (*Blue Sheet* 1991).

Misconduct

As bad as conflicts of interest are, they do not, in themselves, constitute misconduct. Conflicts of interest, either potential or real, may endanger the outcome of the scientific endeavor but are not *willful* destruction of the truth. Scientific misconduct is the purposeful falsification of scientific data or other information to distort the facts; only one master is present—self-interest. It is much less difficult to determine that overt fraud has occurred than to define wrongdoing in conflict of interest (Petersdorf 1989).

Whether egregious carelessness, especially in a senior investigator, is misconduct is a difficult and controversial issue. Further, the distinction between conflict of interest and fraud may not be as sharp as we would like to think. C. P. Snow, for example, noted, "The only ethical principle which has made science possible is that the truth shall be told all the time. If we do not penalise false statements made in error, we open up the way, don't you see, for false statements by intention. And of course a false statement of fact, made deliberately, is the most serious crime a scientist can commit" (Snow 1959). Regardless of this dilemma, misconduct is not further addressed in this volume.

Conflict of Commitment

Conflict of interest is also quite different from conflict of commitment; the latter deals, for example, with deciding whether an academician is fulfilling institutional obligations while under competing demands. This issue has been fully addressed by the Association of American Medical Colleges, which suggested the following for academic faculty members (Ad Hoc Committee on Misconduct and Conflict of Interest in Research 1989):

1. Assure that research, teaching, and public service obligations to the academic institution are fully met.

2. Abide by restrictions on the type and amount of outside activity as determined by the academic institution, or by subsequent agreements between faculty and the university or hospital administration.
3. Abide by commitments of effort as specified in contractual research agreements and grant applications.

As an example, most universities limit consultantships by faculty who have on-campus research sponsored by the same company. The consultantship takes on the flavor of a "salary supplement" if the investigator is paid both by the university and by the company to perform the same work, creating a conflict that is more a conflict of commitment than an abuse of science. This issue is further discussed in Chapter 6. The federal government, for its own employees, strictly prohibits "receiving compensation from two separate sources for the same job" (Rasinski 1987).

Conflicts in Basic and Clinical Research

If conflict of interest is always bad but is also inevitable, then how can one control it (Chapter 10) without strangling the highly successful biomedical industry (Chapter 3) and, worse, slowing progress in disease prevention and amelioration? In biomedical research, the most common approach to limiting the regulatory process has been to emphasize the control of conflict of interest in clinical rather than basic studies.[*]

In considering the logic of emphasizing control over clinical studies, one must first establish what is *not* accomplished by such a tactic. There is no evidence that conflict of interest is less destructive to the basic scientific endeavor than to the clinical. The rigidification of control of clinical investigation, therefore, is not with the aim of "cleaning up the dirtiest part of biomedical science." It is, rather, that emphasizing control at the clinical level addresses society's most vulnerable aspect of biomedical research—the final steps before a product (or a process) is licensed for widespread use with innocent and unsuspecting patients. The rationale for controlling research bias at the clinical trial level, therefore, has little or nothing to do with science per se, but rather with the impact of science on society. Let us further consider the bearable control of conflicts of interest at the basic and clinical levels.

[*]In describing the nature of the studies, some prefer other dichotomous terms such as *evaluative versus fundamental* or *medicine versus science*. I think *clinical versus basic*, while oversimplified, is the most descriptive.

Control of conflict of interest in the basic laboratory, while theoretically possible, is usually quite impractical as "the nature of the research and its susceptibility to scrutiny by nonscientists are dramatically different from clinical trials" (Institute of Medicine 1989). Scientists are quite idiosyncratic in the ways they organize their laboratories, their experiments, and their data. To "watchdog" fundamental studies would require teams of scientists (of the highest caliber, of course) continuously to sort through complex data files on endless experiments (Institute of Medicine 1989). Further, the yield would be low and often controversial. It is much more practical to rely on the present system of *verification* of research in different laboratories. In basic studies—to a much greater degree than in clinical trials—replication is a reliable and pragmatic approach to verify reported results (Snow 1959). Basic studies do not in themselves lead to widespread patient exposure, even though they are the fundament on which clinical trials are based. When untruth does occur in basic studies, not only is it generally easier to uncover, but also the damage is less severe than in a clinical study.

Clinical studies, on the other hand, are the final common pathway to widespread human use. The studies are expensive in both time and money and may be virtually impossible to replicate. Therefore, untruth is harder to uncover than in clinical trials in basic studies, and the societal impact is much greater. As noted by Relman (1989), "later work by others will probably correct any errors resulting from these biases but not before damage has been done by the dissemination of misleading clinical information." The British agree, noting that "spectacular failures in the physical sciences are unlikely to harm the individual, but the obscene damage to countless patients resulting from the application of treatments based on experience and intuition are countless" (Baum 1983); that "it is undesirable for a physician to have any personal financial interest in studies carried out on patients under his/her care" (Wells 1987); and that "physicians responsible for the care of the patients or subjects in these studies should not have a significant financial interest in the company or organization" (Wells 1987).

The potential magnitude of the problem is not trivial. In 1988, 37 percent of the members of the American Federation for Clinical Research (1990) reported that they received pharmaceutical support for at least part of their research. In an attempt to deal with this issue, some investigators have recognized the potential conflicts of interest that a pharmaceutical company has in providing financial support for clinical trials, and they recommended a "code of practice" for industry behavior (Hampton and Julian 1987).

A worse problem is that one study (Davidson 1986) suggested that studies sponsored by pharmaceutical companies are more likely to favor the new therapy than studies supported by a mutual source (Figure 7.1). In an analysis of 107 trials, in which 71 percent favored the new therapy, 43 percent were funded by pharmaceutical companies. Of the 31 trials favoring traditional therapy, only 13 percent (4 trials) were supported by a pharmaceutical company. Although the authors of this study noted that many reasons other than investigator bias may explain these observations, their findings are reason for concern. In fact, "in no case was a therapeutic agent manufactured by the sponsoring company found to be inferior to an alternative product manufactured by another company" (Davidson 1986).

The use of the clinical/basic dichotomy as a paradigm for conflict of interest control is controversial. In its favor, it limits the high-scrutiny areas of conflict of interest to a small fraction of the total research enterprise by concentrating on the scientific areas that are most societally sensitive. It frees up most areas of research (notably basic laboratories) to police themselves, just as is current practice. Against this concept is the erroneous implication that conflict of interest is more detrimental to clinical science than to basic investigation. Also, restriction of clinical conflict of interest singles out one group of scientists for special bureaucratic control. Worse, this control would be exerted on clinical investigators, long an endangered species (Wyngaarden 1979).

Figure 7.1. In this retrospective analysis, 107 trials in five leading medical journals were analyzed with regard to outcome and source of funding. Pharmaceutically funded studies were much less likely to favor traditional therapy, as compared to new therapy.

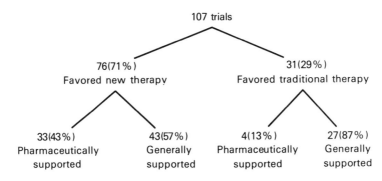

Source: Davidson 1986.

INDUSTRY AND THE TRUTH-SEEKING PROCESS

What are the motivations of industry? First, the people who run and work for companies are no more or less ethical than any other group of ambitious and hard-working professionals. One is unable to discern any difference in ethical standards between colleagues in industry and colleagues in academia; a spectrum exists in each, reflecting the normally distributed population.

Second, industry wants the truth. A company must, in spite of its high hopes for a potential product, be fully aware of whether the product is effective and/or harmful. The company's fundamental approach to science is, according to Bloch, "antithetical to biased reporting or interpretation of research results" (Washington Fax, 1989). Only a company armed with the facts can make a reasonable decision regarding future studies and marketing, as the "truth will out" just as soon as the product is tried on enough patients. Much better that the company learns as early as possible about the limitations of its product than to discover later that a serious defect will harm both the patients and the company that produced it.

A corollary of this need for the company to discover the truth is the need for truth at all levels in the development of a new product. In the development of a new drug, for example, management is dependent on the absolute candor—not to mention quality—of the basic pharmacologist who says the drug is active, of the toxicologist who says the drug is nontoxic (or just how toxic), and of the clinician who says that the drug is safe in studies on human volunteers. In between are dozens of other investigators and technicians who must, with great veracity, convey the data about their studies on the new drug. The data culminate in the controlled clinical trial in human patients, in which the industry's clinical team is entirely dependent on accurate and complete studies from all the scientists who preceded them in the project. Absolute veracity is expected by each of the scientific contributors.

The problem in industry is not, therefore, the company as a whole, or the chain of accurate experiments required to market a product. The problem arises when *individuals* within the company begin to become attached to their product. This attachment can be quite strong and occurs for two reasons. First, the industry investigator may begin to believe in the intrinsic value of the product and may feel strongly that the product is a good one—for both the company and the patients suffering the relevant disorder; the individual's judgment on the various studies, or on which studies should and should not be performed, may then become biased. This belief also comes, in part, from a long-term association with the product and the fear of "wasted years" if it is not successfully marketed. The second reason that an industry investigator may become attached to a product is the desire to be on a winning team; teams that develop successful products are often rewarded by the industry, even though other, equally scientifically sound groups, may have worked just as hard but were not so lucky.

The advantage to the product of having a strong advocate in the company is that, especially in the final clinical push, zeal is very helpful in driving the product through the maze of clinical investigations and approvals required for marketing. The *dis*advantage, however, lies in the infectious enthusiasm of the industry scientist who may convey to the academic investigator that "I know this product is safe and effective." The academician is thereby placed in a difficult position of having to say, "I promise you a good study but I don't promise that your product will prove marketable." Rarely, such a statement may suggest to the industry clinician a lack of interest on the part of the academician and may cause the biased industry clinician to look elsewhere for a different and "more enthusiastic" investigator. Although such behavior on the part of the industry investigator, therefore, can clearly be destructive to the truth-seeking process, most companies recognize this dilemma by having multiple persons involved in the evaluation process.

REFERENCES

Ad Hoc Committee on Misconduct and Conflict of Interest in Research. 1989. *Association of American Medical Colleges.* Washington, D.C.

American Federation for Clinical Research. 1990. Guidelines for avoiding conflict of interest. *Clinical Research,* 38: 239–40.

Baum, M. 1983. The controlled trial and the advance of reliable knowledge. *British Medical Journal,* 287: 1216–7.

Bible: Authorized (King James) Version. Daniel 1:12–15 and Matthew 6:24.

The Blue Sheet. 1991, AMA to revise ethical guidelines for drug marketing. May 15, p. 4.

Bray, D. M. 1990. Conflict of interest: A principal business officer's perspective. *SRA Journal,* Winter, pp. 13–18.

Byar, D. P. 1976. Randomized clinical trials. *New England Journal of Medicine,* 295: 74–80.

The Cardiac Arrhythmia Suppression Trial (CAST) Investigators. 1989. Preliminary Report: Effect of encainide and flecainide on mortality in a randomized trial of arrhythmia suppression after myocardial infarction. *New England Journal of Medicine,* 321(6): 406–12.

Council of the American Association of University Professors and the American Council on Education. 1964. *A Joint Statement: On Preventing Conflicts of Interest in Government-Sponsored Research at Universities.* Washington, D.C.

Council Report. 1990. Conflicts of interest in medical center/industry research relationships. *Journal of the American Medical Association*, 263: 2790–3.

Davidson, R. A. 1986. Source of funding and outcome of clinical trials. *Journal of General Internal Medicine*, 3: 155–8.

Hampton, J. R., and Julian, D. C. 1987. Role of the pharmaceutical industry in major clinical trials. *Lancet*, 2: 1258–9.

Institute of Medicine. 1989. *IOM Report of a Study on the Responsible Conduct of Research in the Health Sciences Clinical Research*, 37: 179–91.

Meinert, C. L. 1986. *Clinical Trials Design, Conduct, and Analysis*. New York: Oxford University Press.

Merton, R. 1973. The normative structure of science. *The Sociology of Science*, 267–78.

Monahan, J., and Bejtlich, N. 1989. NSF creates committee on openness in science. Washington Fax. June 20.

Northrup, F. S. C. 1983. *The Logic of the Sciences and the Humanities*. Woodbridge, Connecticut: Ox Bow Press.

Palca, J. 1989. NIH grapples with conflict of interest. *Ethics in Science*, 245: 23.

Passamani, E. 1991. Clinical trials—are they ethical? *The New England Journal of Medicine*, 324(22): 1589–91.

Petersdorf, R. G. 1989. A matter of integrity. *Academic Medicine*, 64: 119–23.

Physicians' Desk Reference. 1989. Oradell, New Jersey: Medical Economics.

Physicians' Desk Reference. 1991. Oradell, New Jersey: Medical Economics.

Pocock, S. J. 1983. *Clinical Trials: A Practical Approach*. New York: Wiley.

Porter, R. J. 1990. Preface. *Controlled Clinical Trials in Neurological Disease*. Boston: Kluwer Academic.

Rasinski, D. C. 1987. *Conflicts of Interest*: A DM&S Perspective. Long Beach, California: Veterans Administration Medical Center. Veterans Administration Department of Medicine and Surgery, IL 10-87-29.

Rawlins, M. D. 1984. Doctors and the drug makers. *Lancet*, August 4, pp. 276–8.

Relman, A. S. 1989. Economic incentives in clinical investigation. *New England Journal of Medicine*, 320: 933–4.

Report of the Royal College of Physicians. 1986. The relationship between physicians and the pharmaceutical industry. *Journal of the Royal College of Physicians of London*, 20: 235–42.

Rouse, W. H. D. 1956. *Great Dialogues of Plato*. New York: The New American Library.

Sabean, P. 1989. Conflict of interest survey results highlight reluctant support ambiguity and technology transfer concerns. *Washington Fax*, November 30.

Snow, C. P. 1959. *The Search*. New York: Charles Scribner's Sons.

Wells, F. 1987. Promotion by the drug companies: The industry replies. *Journal of the Royal College of Physicians of London*, 37: 271.

Wheelwright, P. 1951. *Wheelwright's Aristotle*. New York: Odyssey.

Wyngaarden, J. B. 1979. The clinical investigator as an endangered species. *New England Journal of Medicine*, 301: 1254–9.

8 • Conflict of Interest in Research: Personal Gain—The Seeds of Conflict

Roger J. Porter

THE FUNDAMENTAL MOTIVATING FACTORS

What factors motivate persons to become scientists and investigators? Also, what causes these investigators to pursue their work, often with a vigor and dedication that astonishes their non-scientific counterparts in the work force? This chapter examines the fundamental factors that motivate scientists, beginning with the most pure—curiosity—and ending with the least pure—pecuniary gain (Figure 8.1).

Curiosity

Curiosity is the fundament of science. The desire to know more and the active search for truth are the purest of motivating factors. For example, the United States recently placed a billion-dollar telescope in orbit so that we might be able to see further and more clearly (even if it does not work very well); there is no obvious altruistic benefit and no apparent pecuniary gain. We are curious about the universe in which we live. Curiosity is closely allied to the truth-seeking process. Curiosity, therefore, is not only a motivating force that is highly characteristic of scientists but also a force that has no biasing potential.

Whether curiosity alone is a sufficient driving force for most scientists is dubious. In most cases, more tangible personal gain is required to keep science in motion.

Figure 8.1. The forces that motivate scientists.

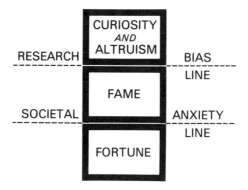

Note: Scientists have several motivations for undertaking investigations in search of the truth. The most objective motivations, with the least investigator bias, are curiosity and altruism. The quest for recognition (fame) is less objective but almost universally tolerated. Pecuniary personal gain (fortune) for the conduct of an experiment can be a powerful counterforce to the truth-seeking process and is viewed by society with considerable suspicion.

Altruism

The desire to improve the world and the plight of its human inhabitants is a motivating factor for many of the most dedicated scientists. It is no longer difficult to see the healing potential of even the most basic biomedical research. Molecular geneticists uncover genes that provide important clues to definitive therapy. Basic pharmacologists manipulate molecules to make better drugs. Clinical investigators test these new drugs to see whether their patients improve. Gratification now extends to biomedical scientists at all levels.

Altruism is, in general, unbiased in its effect on the truth-seeking effort. Occasionally, "the desire to do good" may overwhelm the "desire to know" and may cause the scientist to anticipate the results of an experiment, thus introducing bias, but such events are probably uncommon.

There are those who claim that altruism is nonexistent. "Mother Theresa just wants to go to heaven," say they. Although this extreme view is almost certainly in error, it is, in fact, doubtful that altruism—indeed even when combined with curiosity—is sufficient to drive the scientific machine that we know today.

Fame

Personal gain becomes much more tangible when we consider the array of acknowledgments available for scientific accomplishments. The desire for recognition is, in general, highly respected. Although fame is the crass, extreme end of the recognition spectrum, it is merely one end of a continuum that begins with a modest scientific poster in an obscure part of a scientific meeting. Virtually all scientists want recognition for their work, and the search for fame is not usually considered a conflict of interest. Recognition is, instead, considered a useful motivating factor to make the scientist work hard to contribute to our knowledge (Relman 1989).

The issue, however, is complex. To be credited with "being first" to make an important scientific discovery is to obtain valuable academic currency. Although the scientific community—at least in the abstract—discourages hasty experiments or premature publishing by those who hope to become famous, the penalties are not great; this behavior (and the resultant errors) are considered only slightly out-of-bounds. Most often, the errors are simply corrected and then ignored by the community unless the scientist gets a reputation for frequent mistakes or if the errors have an adverse impact on innocent persons, such as patients. Indeed, a 1991 article on a new genetic discovery—rushed to publication to meet a competitor—was described, after minor flaws were noted by the editor, as "well within accepted accuracy rates" (Roberts 1991).

Nevertheless, the evidence that the desire for fame has potential for damaging the scientific process is considerable. In clinical research, for example, "the desire for public recognition or a tenured faculty position may exert an undue influence on the results" (Council report 1990). The source of this problem lies in the need for *positive studies* in one's academic career—that is, studies that prove that a hypothesis is correct and meaningful. It is very difficult for young investigators to climb the standard ladders of academia if all they have proven is that particular experiments "don't work." Likewise, the need for "positive results" extends to senior investigators who wish national and international recognition for their scientific achievements. Indeed, the most famous investigators are those who provide the greatest insights into their science; the mechanism for achieving this fame is a carefully designed experiment that leads to new knowledge. Only rarely does a negative study provide such insight. If the search for recognition drives the investigator to seek positive studies, then the inevitable hope is that the experiment will yield the expected results; personal gain thereby becomes a driving force on the scientific process. The search for fame is a motivation that is quite different, therefore, from curiosity; the latter is neutral to the experimental outcome and therefore more "scientifically pure," whereas the former may lead to bias.

However, the desire for fame may also serve as a potent force to motivate scientists to work hard at their profession. Whether one speaks of a graduate student working late at night to obtain recognition for scientific insight and productivity or of a senior scientist driving a team toward the Nobel prize, all agree that the desire for recognition is intense, perhaps related to the desire for power, and that great numbers of remarkable scientific accomplishments derive from this energy. Ironically, this same motivator may also yield greater potential for bias; some investigators even think that the desire for fame is more intense and has greater biasing potential than the desire for money.

Before leaving the concept of fame and moving on to fortune, it is important to recognize the inevitable relationship between the two. In many fields, fortune leads to fame. In science, more typically, fame leads to fortune. Even though fortune is usually not measured in hundreds of thousands of dollars for most investigators, it may be measured, for example, in the number of all-expense-paid business-class transatlantic invitations that are received. Alternatively, it may be a more rapid academic climb, with increased remuneration a natural consequence. The desire for fame is inextricably bound to the desire for fortune. This dual concern regarding conflict of interest in science has been addressed by the *Journal of the American Medical Association* (*JAMA*). In attempting to limit the conflicts of its referees (who largely determine what will be published by this prestigious journal), it noted, "The Journal believes, therefore, that the term *conflict of interest* should apply not only to the possibility of financial gain for referees, but also to other, though less easily measurable, interests beyond the financial, such as the possibility of otherwise unmerited gains in priority of publication, personal recognition, career advancement, increased power, or enhanced prestige" (Southgate 1987).

Fortune

The most societally sensitive factor that motivates scientists to work hard is money. Therefore, its potential for biasing the scientific process is great. "It is difficult enough for the most conscientious researchers to be totally unbiased about their own work, but when an investigator has an economic interest in the outcome of the work, objectivity is even more difficult" (Relman 1989). Pecuniary gain comes in all sizes and forms. It is convenient to divide pecuniary gain into gifts, expenses, honoraria, consultantships, royalties, and equity.

Gifts

Most discussions about gifts have been related *not* to research but to clinical practice. "Gifts, hospitality or subsidies offered by medical equipment, pharmaceutical or other manufacturers or distributors ought not to be accepted if acceptance would influence the objectivity of clinical judgment," says the American College of Physicians (1989). How one is to measure such influence is unstated. Gifts, especially small gifts called "reminder items" (Table 8.1), are common in both medicine and science, and these are usually given by a company to enhance its name recognition rather than to influence directly a specific person or a project. While it may be useful to have an extra umbrella or two from a pharmaceutical company, the relationship between small gifts and scientific bias at first seems somewhat remote. Unfortunately, it is not clear that the size of the gift is directly correlated to the effect on the recipient, and some suggest that the value of such trinkets is in the securing of individual relationships, with subtle implications for future obligations (Chren, Landefeld, and Murray 1989; Weiss 1989). At some scientific meetings, small gifts are so common that attendees are also given bags in which to carry them. Books, pens, mementos, pointers, hats, and clocks are all part of the standard fare of commercial scientific exhibits. To the cardiovascular world, at least, receipt of small gifts is "acceptable practice" (Conti et al. 1990). The Council on Ethical and Judicial Affairs of the American Medical Association (AMA) recommended that such items be "related to the physician's work (e.g., pens and notepads)" (Council on Ethical and Judicial Affairs of the American Medical Association 1991).

Some gifts are both expensive and educational. One leading pharmaceutical company, CIBA-GEIGY, subsidizes the distribution of its highly respected clinical symposia and the CIBA collection volumes to physicians; these two publications account for $5.4 million (K. Kernan, personal communication, 1991) of the $6.5 million in gifts given by the company in 1988 (Table 8.1, Column 3).

Large gifts may be less common in the investigative world than in the clinical world. All-expenses-paid trips to a resort for physicians to hear about the merits of a specific drug may cause them to be more inclined to use the company's drug in clinical practice, but such gifts are likely to disappear in the wake of recent recommendations by the aforementioned AMA Council, which eschew acceptance of travel and lodging just to attend a conference (Council on Ethical and Judicial Affairs of the American Medical Association 1991).

Table 8.1. Symposia, Reminders, Gifts, and Honoraria, 1988

Symposia		Reminder Items		Gifts		Honorarial Expenses (faculty and attendee)	
MS&D	$18,861,615	Pfizer	$9,102,298	Ciba-Geigy	$6,465,691	Abbott	$4,916,396
Ciba-Geigy	15,343,941	SmithKline	7,400,000	B-W (b)	5,250,000	Lederle	3,900,000
Lilly	8,890,800	Lilly	5,109,000	Lederle	2,739,935	B-W	2,600,000
Abbott	5,599,276	MS&D	5,105,000	Upjohn	2,204,489	Bristol-Myers	2,498,492
Merrell Dow	5,206,186	J&J	3,967,511	Syntex	1,633,300	Lilly	2,387,750
Searle	5,186,667	Warner-Lambert	2,809,331	Searle	1,287,461	Merrell Dow	909,271
Pfizer	4,820,000	Ciba-Geigy	2,735,343	Roche	1,059,448	Pfizer	900,000
SmithKline	3,710,800	Roche	2,575,130	Bristol-Myers	1,059,000	J&J	520,327
Upjohn	3,532,000	Abbott	2,426,962	Lilly	1,041,000	Ciba-Geigy	377,560
Lederle	2,900,000	Wyeth-Ayerst	2,347,730	J&J	387,082	Searle	331,060 +
Roche	2,657,233	Searle	2,200,861	Warner-Lambert	314,518	Roche	221,768 +
B-W	2,600,000	Syntex	2,107,763	Merrell Dow	212,338	Upjohn	69,000 +
Wyeth-Ayerst	2,363,534	Merrell Dow	2,084,975	Norwich	126,528	Norwich	56,500
Warner-Lambert	2,128,449	Lederle	2,000,000	Abbott	55,985	MS&D	ND
J&J	1,034,605	Norwich	1,518,030	SmithKline	16,180	SmithKline	ND
Syntex	739,999	Bristol-Myers	703,320	MS&D	3,238	Syntex	ND
Norwich	354,500	B-W	600,000	Pfizer	0	Warner-Lambert	ND
Bristol-Myers	ID	Upjohn	ND	Wyeth-Ayerst	(a)	Wyeth-Ayerst	ND

ND = no data; ID = Incomplete data; (a) Included in reminder item total. (b) Includes amounts for continuing education and donations.

Note: This table was compiled by the Congressional Research Service for hearings held by Senator Edward Kennedy on December 11–12, 1991. Symposia are the expenses of educating physicians and other medical persons, exclusive of personal expenses for the faculty and of the attendees (fourth column). Gifts (third column) are heterogeneous and do not include small reminder items (second column). Some of these data, compiled by the Congressional Research Service, have been challenged; see, for example, rebuttal letter from Burroughs Wellcome Co (Hearing, Kennedy, 101-1217, pp. 16–7).

Source: The Blue Sheet, January 2, 1991. Reprinted with permission from F.D.C. Reports, Inc.

Such gifts are less obvious for clinical investigators. Nonetheless, clinical investigators are usually well treated by companies that depend on them, and potential difficulties remain, especially when the investigators and the company staff become emotionally attached to each other. Investigators may wish to please the company that has treated them so well, and they may interpret their role in this relationship as one that requires them to attempt to provide a positive study.

Travel to a Meeting

The next pecuniary gain to be considered is a long-time favorite, the company-sponsored trip by the investigator to a scientific meeting. Some scientists are dependent on such sponsorship to attend the various meetings, and without such support, attendance might suffer somewhat. Typically, the investigator is permitted by the company to attend a limited number of meetings, all of which are relevant to the studies undertaken; some may include presentations of the work performed under company sponsorship. Is funding for travel to a meeting a perquisite? One might say, quite correctly, that meetings are hard work and a necessary part of information exchange. On the whole, however, meetings present a pleasant break in the academic routine and are generally viewed as one of the more desirable tasks of an academician. When the meeting faculty is chosen by the pharmaceutical company, some of the company's academic investigators are almost always included as speakers. It is worth observing the British recommendations with regard to meeting expenses: "Support from the pharmaceutical industry for scientific and educational meetings is invaluable, but sponsorship of speakers and attenders should be decided independently and payment should not be arranged directly between a pharmaceutical company and a physician. Companies should be encouraged to make their donations for these purposes to the organizing committees and proper acknowledgement of their support should be made. If a company offers travel funds in the form of scholarships, its name may be indicated but applications for such support should be submitted to the organizers and the selection made independently by them and not by the company" (Report of Royal College of Physicians 1986). The AMA Council has similar recommendations (Council on Ethical and Judicial Affairs of the American Medical Association 1991).

Honoraria

More serious pecuniary gain begins with honoraria, in which a company actually pays the academician for a lecture, an article, or some other product. An *honorarium* is "a reward, usually for services, on which custom or propriety forbids a price to be set" (Webster's Seventh New Collegiate Dictionary 1965); the ostensible distinction is from a "fee," in which the charge is relatively fixed. Honoraria can be given to academicians in innumerable ways and in remarkably different settings.

Although honoraria have received a bad name (they are, at the moment, almost altogether banned in the U.S. federal government), many represent reasonable compensation for work performed. The danger for science comes when companies give honoraria to their active investigators; such highly desirable honoraria typically range from one hundred to several thousand dollars. They may cause the academician to lose objectivity in the scientific endeavor; the desire to please the company may influence the scientific outcome or the interpretation of the results. The potential for conflict of interest was raised in one recent example, in which a physician received research funding from private industry but also "received more than $50,000 each year in honoraria from private industry, most of it in the form of speaking fees from three of the pharmaceutical companies involved in the studies" (Committee on Government Operations, U.S. House of Representatives 1990).

For the average citizen, at least, it is difficult to imagine that such remuneration would not endear the companies to the investigator. Interestingly enough, most (though not all) proposals for controlling conflict of interest do not proscribe honoraria. One of the most widely quoted voluntary guidelines, for example, requires only annual reporting of "the participation of investigators in educational activities supported by companies" (Healy 1989). Another, Harvard Medical School, considers honoraria "routinely allowable" (Harvard University Faculty of Medicine 1990). The American Federation for Clinical Research, on the other hand, considers honoraria a source of income which has a "potential for conflict of interest" (American Federation for Clinical Research 1990). Honoraria are dearly beloved, especially for speeches. Talking is fun; to be paid for it is heaven.

So what are reasonable honoraria guidelines, for example, for lectures? Bricker suggested that

> such activities should be accepted as services warranting remuneration only if the entire program has a bona fide educational character and is not primarily promotional; if the mention of any commercial product by name is either incidental or occurs in a scientific context without exaggeration or unbalanced claims; if the presentation is based on valid scientific data or a substantial clinical experience that justifies it; and if the honorarium

is proportional to the work performed, and the travel expenses are not lavish (the fact that a payment markedly exceeds customary levels should be made evident to the audience during the program). Lectures or seminars that are offered as part of a full-time or part-time contractual arrangement with a medical-service company should also include the disclosure of the relationship. (Bricker 1989)

Laudable though these restrictions are, they do not address the degree to which honoraria are acceptable if an investigator is simultaneously studying a company's product and lecturing in educational programs sponsored by the same company. In an effort to address this issue more directly, the Parkinson Study Group (PSG), a highly productive group of clinical investigators, strictly limits honoraria:

Certain activities with "involved companies" are not considered to be a conflict-of-interest. But no personal compensation shall accrue to the PSG member for these activities, although the intended compensation can be directed to a public charity, scientific society or to the member's department, university or hospital, including an academic account administered by the PSG member. These activities must be disclosed annually by December 31st to the Steering Committee. These activities include: (a) serving as an educator, e.g., giving a lecture or speaking in a panel discussion at a forum sponsored by an "involved company"; (b) participating in research activities unrelated to the study drug or product, and supported by the "involved company." (Parkinson Study Group 1990)

The distinction between consultantship and honoraria becomes blurred when honoraria reach large sums, with frequent interchange between academician and the company. Indeed, the editor of *JAMA* notes that "honoraria are a big problem; obviously the word is a euphemism." He then noted that to provide full disclosure "we would consider putting honoraria in parentheses the next time we revise our instructions to authors" (Blue Sheet 1989a).

Consultantships

One step up from honoraria is for the academician to be a consultant to the company. Consultantships are likewise heterogeneous; they may involve one or two days per year at less than $1000 per day or may involve many days, with accumulated fees of tens of thousands of dollars per year. Many academicians feel that honoraria are acceptable but that consultantships involve a special commitment to industry; consultantships are sometimes perceived, therefore, as associated with diminished academic purity.

Curiously, whereas industry is not (except at the marketing level) needful of paying honoraria, it is continuously in need of sophisticated advice. "We would be at a loss if we could not get consultants from academia," noted one pharmaceutical company vice president (Blue Sheet 1989b). Another executive stated, "industry couldn't be profitable without a strong academic connection" (Panem 1984). Indeed, one might argue that the current success of the U.S. pharmaceutical industry is directly related to the extraordinary expertise in biomedicine, an expertise largely created by the federal government—especially in basic science. Consultation with industry may provide pecuniary gain to the academician, but the societal importance derives from the critical role such consultants play for the industry.

Consultants are more interested in company policy than are those who take an occasional honorarium. Indeed, if one perceives that a consultant is (for a brief period, at least) part of the company itself, the consultant should share in the need to be part of the truth-seeking chain in the company's research effort (discussed in Chapter 7). The consultant may even become hyperconservative; if risks are not recommended, the consultant has a smaller probability of eventually being embarrassed by a suggestion. Clearly there is nothing wrong with being a company consultant. The danger to science occurs when the consultant is also the investigator; such arrangements have been discouraged for clinical research (Healy 1989).

Royalties
Pecuniary return from inventions is in a special position in the system of personal gains. To receive royalties on intellectual property rights is a very natural and normal part of a free-market society. Unfortunately, royalties are usually a direct function of sales of the product, and these present a tangible conflict of interest for any inventor who is also part of the evaluation process. Suppose, for example, a clinician invents a device that promises some market potential, all rights to the device are sold to a company (large or small), in exchange for royalties, and then the clinician wishes personally to evaluate the product in a clinical trial. The two masters are more than apparent. When such a situation arises, the company may wish to hire the inventor as a consultant but to contract with other scientists to conduct the needed clinical studies. This should allow the expertise of the inventor to be reflected, for example, in appropriate protocol design but preclude the royalty recipient from participating in the actual evaluation process.

Equity

"Owning stock in a company at the same time one is conducting research, the results of which can affect the stock's value, creates the potential for bias, whether intended or not" (Lichter 1989). *Equity* (stocks, stock options, etc.) is controversial as an agent of conflict of interest, not because the holding of equity theoretically creates a potential for biasing science—which it obviously does—but because of the heterogeneity of the size and relative influence of equity holdings. The potential for equity to interfere with the truth-seeking scientific process is complex but is best summarized by describing two settings, which represent the extreme possibilities.

The first is with a small product and a large company. When an investigator is studying a product for a large company, in which the product is unlikely to have, even if successful, a large impact on the company or its stock, the potential for conflict of interest is not great. Unfortunately, (1) it is not always possible to predict the ultimate value of a product, and (2) it is not always possible to predict the expectations of the investigator, who is very often emotionally attached to the product. The investigator's expectation of good results for the product, even though the product will not have a major impact on the company, can be destructive to the truth-seeking process.

The second example is the opposite extreme. Relative to the company size, the product looms very large. In start-up companies, it may be the only product; the entire company may rise or fall on the clinical applicability and marketability of the product. An example of how conflict of interest may interfere with the truth-seeking effort under such circumstances is given in Chapter 9 (the Boston "eyedrops" story). Most venture capital investors will not permit the inventor-owner of the company to be the sole evaluator of the product; the potential for conflict of interest is simply too great to make such an evaluation credible.

In most circumstances, therefore, it is questionable whether the clinical investigator of a product should have equity in a company that may financially benefit from a successful investigation. In some cases, the product's limited potential in a large company may limit the likelihood that the holding of equity would be a problem; in other cases, the danger of conflict of interest may be considerable and, as noted by Frommer et al., "Some research may have a significant impact on even very large companies" (Frommer et al. 1990). Some universities prohibit faculty from having equity interest in a company that supports on-campus research by that faculty member (Johns Hopkins University School of Medicine 1989).

When defining prohibitions on equity, most (including the federal government) eliminate interests "over which the investigator has no control, such as mutual funds and blind trusts" (Healy 1989).

OTHER MOTIVATING FACTORS: INDIRECT AND NONPECUNIARY PERSONAL GAINS

Not all gains that can be derived in science fall neatly into the categories of fame, gifts, and monetary accumulation. Other kinds of gains, often more indirect and subtle, can be equally desirable to the investigator. In most cases, the gains can ultimately be related back to the four fundamental motivating factors—curiosity, altruism, fame, and fortune. Sorting out which motivation is actually most important in these indirect benefits is often impossible.

Laboratory Benefits

The argument is often made that indirect gains such as the funding of studies themselves are for the scientist's *laboratory* and not for the investigator's personal gains. If one considers the motivating factors important to scientists, however, it is clear that scientists and their laboratories are inextricable; what is good for the laboratory is good for the scientist. Again, such gains are usually to the benefit of all concerned and are by no means evil in themselves. Some of these gains, which relate to university resources, are discussed in Chapter 6.

Nonindustry Resources

When industry contracts with the university to accomplish its needed research (Chapter 6), included in the agreement are provisions for utilizing university facilities, for which the company pays both direct and indirect (overhead) costs. Conflicts do not usually occur but may arise under some circumstances. For example, investigators may accept large gifts to their academic laboratories instead of signing formal contracts with companies; this procedure may allow these companies to avoid paying indirect costs to the university. These investigators, by oral agreement, accomplish the studies desired by the industry, but the university must pay the overhead for these investigations.

Another, more subtle, example occurs when investigators use funds from a federal grant or some other source to further the research needs of a company, which may have hired these investigators as consultants. In many cases, the use of such facilities and resources is entirely legitimate. In fact, the congressional intent of the Bayh-Dole Act of 1980 was to encourage entrepreneurial exploitation by the universities of new intellectual property or new products derived therefrom. Although it was not the intent of the U.S. Congress that federal research grants to a university be subverted to an industrial subsidy, so long as the original aim of the federal research grant remains intact (i.e., the thrust of the research remains within the original scope of work), the investigator is permitted—encouraged by most universities—to collaborate with industry on the project. Thus, willful changing of the work's scope as specified in the grant, in order to derive personal gain might be considered fraud rather than conflict of interest.

Gains to Senior Scientists

Indirect gains may come to the investigator because of seniority in the laboratory. When junior investigators create valuable intellectual property, the sharing of this value with the senior investigator is usually highly appropriate. When supervision is distant, however, the issue becomes more complex. Unfortunately, as noted by Merton, "the more prominent scientists tend to get the lion's share of recognition" (Merton 1988), even when the originator of the idea is the first author on the publication.

Students

Students may assist in the scientific effort funded by industry. "There is no cheaper, more technologically sound labor than our graduate students," stated one mid-Atlantic university professor (Best 1987). Whether the students benefit from the experience or they are simply exploited varies with the nature of the study and the sensitivity of the investigators. The American Federation for Clinical Research is explicit: "The restrictions involved in industry-sponsored university-based research make it inappropriate for students to participate in these projects" (American Federation for Clinical Research 1990). This point of view may be too rigid but certainly makes clear the anxiety regarding abuse of students. In a survey of 693 graduate students and postdoctoral fellows at six research intensive universities, Gluck et al. (1987) observed the benefits of industrial research and training relationships and concluded that these benefits (such as the availability of funding) outweigh the potential problems. Having thus concluded, however, the authors urged careful university monitoring of (1) delays in publications of research, especially if a trainee's career is dependent on publication, (2) industrial limitation of research topics, (3) requirements for posttraining employment, and (4) the incentive for faculty to use students "for their own financial benefit."

Sharing of Data

Personal gain may also occur when data—usually data that may lead the investigator to fame or fortune—are sequestered rather than shared freely. While some withholding of data, especially before studies are complete, is entirely legitimate and may even be scientifically mandatory (for example, in certain clinical trials), the potential for pecuniary gain from intellectual property has undoubtedly increased the level of secrecy in science. The sequestration may be to only specific scientific colleagues, or it may be general, as to scientific journals; it also may represent only a delay in making public the new information. Some delay is expected to protect patent rights. The omission of key features of scientific data or even distortion of the information presented is less extreme than total secrecy but obviously suboptimal for the advancement of science. Overall, secrecy is often in the service not of science but of personal gain; its legitimacy is therefore limited.

Sharing of Materials

Most of the same arguments that apply to the secrecy of intellectual property also hold for research materials. Valuable materials such as enzymes and molecular probes are commonly shared, but recognition of their potential value in creating new knowledge—and the fear that this will be accomplished by the recipient—has led to a lessening of such sharing. In general, science is at least delayed by such tactics, which are based on the anticipation of personal gain. A consortium of organizations, including the National Institutes of Health and the Pharmaceutical Manufacturers Association, is working to produce a prototype uniform biological material transfer agreement that will minimize the ambiguity of terminology and will expedite material transfers.

CONCLUSION

It is important to recognize that the accumulation of fame and fortune is not evil; on the contrary, it is an integral part of economically successful societies. Furthermore, there is no need to make dire assumptions about the veracity of scientists; indeed, as noted by Harvard University Faculty of Medicine (1990), (1) the vast majority of scientists are honest and conduct their research with the highest standards and integrity, and (2) for the vast majority of cases, self-regulating structures and processes in science are effective. The pursuit of personal gain—in and for itself—is natural and desirable. Personal gain in science is also desirable as long as science is the principal master. Only when personal gain becomes a significant second master—with a separate agenda for the outcome or interpretation of a study—does conflict of interest arise.

In the search for truth, however, specific boundary conditions must be indicated to accomplish the goal of scientific veracity, even though these boundaries limit the classical rewards built into our economic system. Little is likely to be done about the recognition-seeking behavior of scientists; if recognition were to be abolished, there is no doubt that science would fail to advance at anything like its current pace. Society has, however, great anxiety about pecuniary gain interfering with the truth-seeking process; in this arena, guidelines will clearly be required. Finally, as noted in the previous chapter, there is considerable merit to the notion of emphasizing control over conflict of interest in clinical studies and de-emphasizing control in nonclinical investigations.

REFERENCES

American College of Physicians. 1989. American College of Physicians Ethics Manual. Part 1. History, the patient, other physicians. *Annals of Internal Medicine,* 3: 251.

American Federation for Clinical Research. 1990. Guidelines for avoiding conflict of interest. *Clinical Research,* 38: 239.

Bayh–Dole Act of 1980. Public Law 96-517.

Best, D. 1987. Forging a new relationship. *Prepared Foods,* 156: 132.

The Blue Sheet. 1991, January.

The Blue Sheet. 1989a, June. p. 6

The Blue Sheet. 1989b, July. p. 2

Bricker, E. M. 1989. Sounding board: Industrial marketing and medical ethics. *New England Journal of Medicine,* 320: 1690–2.

Chren, M., Landefeld, C. S., and Murray, T. H. 1989. *Journal of the American Medical Association,* 262: 3448–51.

Committee on Government Operations, U.S. House of Representatives. 1990. 19th Report, 101st Congress, 2nd Session. p. 30

Conti, R. C., et al. 1990. Task Force V: The relation of cardiovascular specialists to industry, institutions, and organizations. *Journal of the American College of Cardiology,* 16: 30.

Council on Ethical and Judicial Affairs of the American Medical Association.

1991. Gifts to physicians from industry. *Journal of the American Medical Association*, 265: 501.

Council Report. 1990. Conflicts of interest in medical center/industry research relationships. *Journal of the American Medical Association*, 263: 2790–1.

Frommer, P. L., et al. 1990. Task Force IV: Scientific responsibility and integrity in medical research. *Journal of the American College of Cardiology*, 16: 24–29.

Gluck, M. E., et al. 1987. University-industry relationships in the life sciences: Implications for students and postdoctoral fellows. *Research Policy*, 16: 327–36.

Harvard University Faculty of Medicine. 1990. *Policy on Conflicts of Interest and Commitment*. Cambridge, Massachusetts. p. 7.

Healy, B. 1989. Special report: Conflict-of-interest guidelines for a multicenter clinical trial of treatment after coronary-artery bypass-graft surgery. *New England Journal of Medicine*, 320: 949–51.

Johns Hopkins University School of Medicine. 1989. *Policy on Conflict of Commitment and Conflict of Interest*. Baltimore, Maryland.

Lichter, P. R. 1989. Biomedical research, COI and the public trust. *Ophthalmology*, 96: 575–8.

Merton, R. K. 1988. The Matthew effect in science. *II ISIS*, 79: 606–23.

Panem, S. 1984. *The Interferon Crusade*. Washington, D.C.: Brookings Institution. p. 82

Parkinson Study Group. 1990. *Ethical and Conflict-of-Interest Guidelines for Members of the Parkinson Study Group*.

Relman, A. S. 1989. Economic incentives in clinical investigation. *New England Journal of Medicine*, 320: 933–4.

Report of the Royal College of Physicians. 1986. The relationship between physicians and the pharmaceutical industry. *Journal of the Royal College of Physicians of London*, 20: 239.

Roberts, L. 1991. The rush to publish. *Science*, 251: 260–3.

Southgate, M. 1987. Conflict of interest and the peer review process. *Journal of the American Medical Association*, 258: 1375.

Webster, M. 1965. *Webster's Seventh New Collegiate Dictionary*.

Weiss, T. 1989. Research that the U.S. government is paying for should not be tainted by any possibility of bias. *The Chronicle of Higher Education*, October 4.

9 • Conflict of Interest in Research: Investigator Bias—The Instrument of Conflict

Roger J. Porter

In the conduct of deductive biomedical science, either basic or clinical, scientists are confronted with a question. They then gather all available information on this question and, based on a theory, propose a testable hypothesis. The hypothesis is then tested in an experiment. Scientists carry out the experiment and collect the data, tabulate and analyze the results, and finally put the experiment into perspective with discussion and conclusions, based on both this experiment and other available information. The object of this conduct of science is the accumulation of knowledge. Each hypothesis, experiment, observation, and conclusion is an effort to add, cumulatively, to our understanding of nature. It is, at the very least, a search for the truth about nature (Kneller 1978).

Virtually no one would challenge the notion that science, and the application of the knowledge generated by scientific endeavors, has radically altered the manner in which humans deal with themselves and their environment. Yet much of the scientific process itself is misunderstood by persons who are not directly involved in it and who do not appreciate the pitfalls and limitations of the scientific approach, even considering that science is a "highly variable animal" (Woolgar 1988).

There are, in fact, a startling number of ways in which the aforementioned scientific process fails to achieve its objectives. The question to be asked may be trivial, or it may be too difficult. The hypothesis may be poorly defined or contradictory (Committee on the Conduct of Science, National Academy of Science 1989). The experimental plan may be deficient, or it may be inadequately executed or recorded. Further, the conclusions may be incorrect even though the experiment was properly executed. In spite of the scientists' best efforts, all of the preceding problems occur quite frequently and are, in fact, *expected* in the normal process of searching for the truth. The process of attempting to advance our understanding of nature requires an astonishing tolerance for trial and error.

Errors that result when the process goes awry are considered "honest" errors (except when deliberate fraud occurs) and are clearly normal and necessary. This is not to say that the best scientists do not, in general, originate the best questions, formulate the best hypotheses, design the best experiments, and so on, because the best scientists do exactly that. However, all scientists are at least occasionally liable for the failure of experiments, which, while disappointing, usually adds to the scientist's understanding of the issue; this understanding provides the foundation for the next hypothesis and the next experiment. Nor can one say that all scientific experiments have the potential for obtaining certainty or that science is the only method of seeking truth. Dudley, in a trenchant analysis of "reliable knowledge," suggested, for example, that controlled clinical trials are just one effective method of approaching the truth (Figure 9.1) and that accumulated experience is probably responsible for 80 percent of "what we do and what we do well" (Dudley 1983). Nevertheless, the placement of controlled trials nearest the pole of "certainty" and the placement of "experience" nearest the pole of "ignorance" strongly urge one toward the scientific search for the truth.

Figure 9.1. Continuum of reliability in establishing the truth.

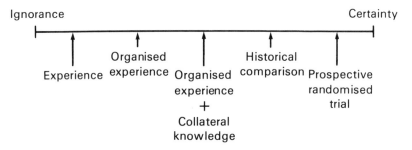

Source: Dudley 1983. Reprinted with permission from the *British Medical Journal,* published by the British Medical Association.

Considering how difficult this truth-seeking process really is, it is not surprising that special scrutiny is provided for one of the weakest aspects of the scientific process—notably, the investigator's desire to have the experiment come out in a predetermined way; this desire and its effects are termed *investigator bias*. The various motivations that may affect the scientist's view of how the experiment "should turn out" are considered at length in the previous chapter. Some of these unconscious motivations may damage the process of science because the *objectivity* needed in seeking truth is compromised. It is noteworthy that—misconduct aside—the only real reason for controlling the conflict of interest in research is investigator bias that arises from personal gain. In other words, if the experiment could be performed in a completely objective manner in the presence of personal gain, conflict of interest in research would not be a problem. Unfortunately, as is demonstrated in the next section of this chapter, bias is the instrument of conflict of interest and must be controlled.

INVESTIGATOR BIAS: GENERAL CONCEPTS

As reviewed in the previous chapter, the desire for acknowledgment for scientific accomplishments in science is, in general, a highly respected goal. Virtually all scientists want recognition for their work, and the search for fame (one end of the recognition spectrum) is not usually considered a conflict of interest. Likewise, all scientists wish to be paid for their work. When pecuniary gain can influence the outcome of a study, however, we call this interference *investigator bias resulting from financial conflicts of interest*.

Investigator bias is the interruption of the ordinarily objective process of science by the injection of the investigator's opinion into the hypothesis-testing effort. This opinion is—in itself—not harmful, is conscious and/or subconscious, is usually based on an intuitive expectation—or hope—about the outcome of the study, and is often partly incorporated into the hypothesis itself. The experiment itself is performed to objectively test the investigator's intuition and therefore must be free of bias. Investigator bias can be inserted at numerous steps in the scientific event, however, and can have a detrimental effect on the truth-seeking effort. The difference in the public health impact from bias in a basic laboratory study versus a clinical trial has been reviewed in Chapter 8. Because bias may be perceived to be different in these two settings, each is considered separately in this chapter.

INVESTIGATOR BIAS IN BASIC RESEARCH

Although bias in clinical research is more studied than bias in the basic laboratory, bias occurs frequently in basic studies and has just as much impact on the research results as might occur in a clinical investigation. Bias may occur at the very beginning of the study in the choosing of an inappropriate question. It may occur in the choice of hypothesis to test, the experiment to be performed, the collection of the data, the evaluation of the data, or the conclusion.

An example is instructive. The following was a real event; details of identification have been deliberately obscured:

> In an outstanding laboratory, an extremely talented and innovative young investigator developed a theory about the nature of the cell membrane, the thin filmlike enclosure that surrounds each cell in the animal body. The theory could be tested, using a little-known biochemical technique which was, in itself, of considerable scientific interest. The young scientist spent many weeks working out the details of the experiment and even more time in its performance. Enthusiasm was high; if the expected and hoped-for outcome of the study was indeed the result, a significant scientific milestone would have been attained. Such a result would have been good for the careers of all those involved in the effort.
>
> The experiment was successful. The hoped-for results were clearly documented in the rats used in the studies. Furthermore, control rats had been used, so that the new positive results were compared to results from rats that had had a different treatment; such controls, which are routine in most good laboratories, gave the required margin of credence to the results. Everyone was elated.
>
> Because of the importance and potential impact of the discovery, however, a senior scientist asked to see the data and to review the experiment with the junior investigator. No flaws were found, but the senior person requested that the study be reconducted as a *blind experiment* (i.e., in a manner in which the investigative team would not know which animals received the experimental treatment and which were the control rats). Although this request made the experiment slightly more difficult to perform, and although publication would necessarily be delayed until the original results were confirmed by the modified experiment, all involved agreed to this replication process requested by the senior scientist. The new experiment would *control for investigator bias,* as the investigators would not know which animal was which until after all the work was finished.
>
> Unfortunately, the newly designed experiment failed to confirm the exciting results of the initial study. Repeated efforts permitted only one

conclusion: the initial study was in error. Even though the hypothesis remained viable, it could not be proven to be true by these experiments. Neither the source of the bias nor the nature of the original errors was ever identified. The studies were eventually discontinued. Disappointment was rife and intense.

What went wrong and why? We know that the investigators who conducted the study were fundamentally honest. Although the desire for fame might have been involved, no personal monetary gain was to be derived from the experiment, which was carried out using federal funds; no proprietary interests were involved. From the usual standpoint of scientific endeavors, the experiment was a typical altruistic search for the truth. The most likely conclusion is that the initial experiment was in some way guided by the investigators to a certain desired outcome; when this guidance was removed by better control of investigator bias, the exciting results could not be duplicated. The initial findings were simply not correct and did not reflect the truth.

In the weeks following the aforementioned disappointment, these investigators designed different studies to tackle different questions, and the process of science moved on. The investigators were painfully educated about the importance of bias control, and some valuable research resources were lost, but otherwise, the experiment had little effect. Even if the original results had been published, relatively minor damage to society would have occurred. To be sure, even more resources might have been wasted by others who attempted, unsuccessfully, to duplicate the results, but the findings would eventually have been discredited and no innocent person (such as patients) were at risk for injury in the process.

Suppose, however, that these same investigators had been working for a pharmaceutical company. Suppose they thought they had discovered an important new drug for a human disease. Would the outcome have been different? Even though the motivation of the scientists was equally intense, the outcome would almost certainly be the same as for the academic scientists. Following the initial success, rigorous internal controls would have been applied to repeat studies. If necessary, and especially for important discoveries, the experiment would be carried out in an entirely separate laboratory to document its outcome (D. Sophia, personal communication, March 1989).

The danger of untruth is most intense when the motivation by the investigator for a desired study outcome is so strong that appropriate control is difficult or even impossible. The worst scenario occurs when the scientist has direct financial interest in the outcome (i.e., when money flows to the investigator if the hoped-for outcome of the study is realized). The studies that are the most likely to be damaging to society are not the basic studies but clinical investigations—where "the public could be put at risk" (Weiss 1989).

INVESTIGATOR BIAS IN CLINICAL RESEARCH

Bias in clinical research is the "unconscious distortion in the selection of patients, collection of data, determination of end points, and final analysis" (Chalmers 1983a). The intrusion of bias in clinical research may also occur at any stage of the scientific process: at inception or in the conclusions or anywhere between (Friedman et al. 1985). Typically, it occurs during the data-collection process, when the term *observer bias* may be used.

An example is instructive. The following, taken from the author's experience (Porter 1988), is typical of epilepsy research in which a high degree of bias control is not included in the study design.

In a clinical trial of a new potential antiepileptic drug, the study was *not blinded* (i.e., both the patient and the doctor knew whether the patient was taking the new compound or taking a placebo). Seizure frequency was the outcome variable: If most of the patients had fewer seizures when taking the new compound than when taking the placebo, the drug would be declared useful and—given sufficient studies—marketed for general use by the 2 million persons with epilepsy in the United States. During an *evaluation period* (i.e., a period during which seizure occurrence—or lack thereof—has a direct effect on the outcome of the trial), the patient had an event at home that was atypical but witnessed by a relative. The investigator was then asked by the staff to decide whether or not this event was or was not a "seizure." This task is often not an easy one, as the investigator must judge purely by the history given by the relative.

Because the investigator knew whether the patient was taking the new compound or taking the placebo, the investigator was in a unique position to influence the trial. By calling the event a "nonseizure" if the patient was on the new compound (or by calling the event a "seizure" if the patient was on the placebo), the study could be biased directly in favor of the new compound. The likelihood of insertion of bias was especially high because of the ambiguity of the nature of the seizurelike event.

Clearly, it is not possible for the investigator to be objective in this kind of decision unless the study is *double blind* (i.e., the patients and the persons involved in the decisions that may unfavorably influence the major goal of the trial are unaware of whether the patient is taking the new compound being tested or the placebo against which the new drug must prove itself). If, in the preceding case, the study were double blind, the investigator could comfortably make the most objective decision regarding the seizurelike event, independent of any desire, conscious or unconscious, to influence the trial with his or her own bias (Porter 1988). It is for good reason that the U.S. Food and Drug Administration (FDA) requires highly controlled studies before consideration for marketing. This is not to say that uncontrolled pilot studies have no value, but merely that most therapies need eventually to be tested in a manner that controls for investigator bias; "the effort to limit and define bias must be assiduous and continuous" (Chalmers et al. 1983a).

In the preceding example, the physician has biased the study in favor of the new drug. The bias was not conscious or malicious but occurred nonetheless. One might ask, Why would the direction of bias favor the new drug? Why not favor the placebo? The answer lies in the nature of clinical trials themselves. All physicians who are conducting a clinical trial of a new drug (or other therapy) are hoping that the new drug will be effective. The reasons for this hope are clear: First, the physicians have a desire to help their patients, and second, everyone wants to be associated with finding something new that works, rather than reporting that a proposed new therapy is ineffective. Even worse, from the standpoint of study bias, everyone else associated with the trial also wants the new drug to work. Not only the physicians but also the nurses, the nurse's aides, the technicians, the patients, the patients' relatives—everyone wants the new drug to be effective and wants to be associated with the discovery of something new and useful for the alleviation of human disease.

The result is that study bias is virtually all in the same direction, which is to suggest that a proposed new therapy is effective when it may not be at all effective. The problem was well analyzed by Chalmers et al. (1983a), who evaluated treatment assignment in 145 clinical trials of the therapy of myocardial infarction (heart attack). He divided the trials into three groups: (1) those in which treatment assignment was highly controlled for bias (i.e., both randomized and blinded), (2) those in which treatment assignment was partly controlled for bias (i.e., randomized but not blinded), and (3) those in which treatment assignment was not controlled for bias (i.e., neither randomized nor blinded). Studies with the highest level of investigator bias control demonstrated a therapy to be effective only 9 percent of the time; studies with some bias control demonstrated a therapy to be effective 24 percent of the time; studies with no bias control demonstrated a therapy to be effective an astonishing 58 percent of the time! From a cynical point of view, the obvious way to prove that a drug is effective is to study it in a poorly designed trial.

The implications of the preceding observations are enormous. If studies that have inadequate bias control are likely to give information that is erroneous, then clinical studies without such bias control may incorrectly conclude that a new drug is effective when, in fact, it is not. Indeed, the inescapable conclusion is that many of the studies reviewed by Chalmers—especially among those in which bias control was inadequate—were simply wrong. Such studies not only fail to contribute to our knowledge but also create erroneous information, which (1) suggests that therapies are effective when they are not (in the extreme, they can injure the patient), (2) falsely heightens patient expectations, and (3) eventually mandates efforts to correct the error with additional, expensive, better-controlled clinical investigations. Thus, even when no direct financial benefits accrue to the investigator, investigator bias seriously flaws experimental research and results.

INVESTIGATOR BIAS AND
WELL-CONTROLLED INVESTIGATIONS

Some investigators who oppose vigorous limitations on pecuniary gains from the performance of research argue that (1) investigator influence on the study outcome is present regardless of financial considerations—the need for recognition is a sufficient driving force, and (2) proper study design can control investigator bias derived from the desire for both fame and fortune.

The truth is not crystal clear. Many would suggest that regardless of the origin of bias, even the best design may not prevent its intrusion into a study. On the other hand, others declare that a rigorously controlled study will prevent such intrusion (although clearly it will not prevent fraud). Two fundamental observations, however, partly negate the latter, more optimistic argument.

First, studies are often not as well controlled as they appear in the protocol. Subtle (and sometimes not so subtle) side effects of a drug under study, for example, can easily unmask the blind in at least some of the patients in the investigation; just a few biased observations derived from such clinical observations can have a critical effect on the outcome, especially of a drug that has marginal utility. If pecuniary gain is added to the need for recognition, investigator bias may become a more potent force; the investigator is even more likely to make erroneous, biased observations. Even the appearance that money can influence the study outcome is unacceptable (Healy 1989).

Second, and closely related to the first observation, the investigators are responsible, after the controlled portion of the study is finished, for the final analysis and interpretation of the data. These analyses and interpretations are at risk for investigator bias, but bias control of such interpretations is difficult; investigators on the same study frequently disagree on the final, critical wording of a manuscript—wording that may greatly influence the interpretation of the study by others. Needless to say, the owner of the product also has a stake in the interpretation of the results, and the risk of bias is heightened when company writers assist in drafting the manuscript (Committee on Labor and Human Resources 1991).

The American Medical Association's Councils on Scientific Affairs and Ethical and Judicial Affairs agreed with this pessimistic view of "design control" of investigator bias: "For the clinical investigator who has an economic interest in the outcome of his or her research, objectivity is especially difficult. Economic incentives may introduce subtle biases into the way research is conducted, analyzed, or reported, and these biases can escape detection by even careful peer review" (Council on Scientific Affairs and Council on Ethical and Judicial Affairs 1990).

In summary, we are influenced by our cultural norms, which suggest that even the appearance of conflict of interest may be socially undesirable. Financial rewards that depend on the outcome of a clinical trial violate these norms much more than the mere accumulation of accolades. Fame—at least in this setting—is a more socially acceptable reward than fortune.

INVESTIGATOR BIAS AND THE BORDERLANDS OF FRAUD

The two previous examples of investigator bias document that subtle—even subconscious—influences can affect the outcome of a scientific study. In both of these cases, however, personal gain was limited to recognition and potential fame for scientific discovery; no monetary personal gain was directly involved. These examples are the most typical of problems of investigator bias, in which the only tangible conflict of interest derives from the desire for fame. What happens when pecuniary reward is involved in the study outcome? In most cases, the science may well progress normally, without undue bias; most investigators are fundamentally honest and seek the truth. On the other hand, clear documentation of how money can mix poorly with clinical science is well shown in the following case, summarized largely from the investigative work of Gosselin (1988):

> A young ophthalmologist with impeccable credentials (including both an M.D. and a Ph.D.) began investigating—along with other colleagues—Vitamin A eye drops for a form of "dry eye," a particularly painful and vexing ophthalmologic problem. The physician-investigators, heavily supported by federal grants, performed a series of initial studies and became impressed by the seeming beneficial effect of the eye drops on patients who were refractory to other treatments. Without publishing definitive scientific data (other than case reports) which could be scrutinized, however, the investigators provided encouraging reports for the lay press. About the same time, the investigators formed a company to take advantage of the new discovery, and stock was sold to enthusiastic investors who anticipated a large return when the product was finally marketed. The investigators reserved three fourths of the stock for themselves. Although later studies had "placebo" controls, the investigators had a direct financial conflict of interest. The outcome of the studies—which they were performing themselves—would directly influence the value of their stock. Monetary personal gain could directly influence and interfere with the truth-seeking process.
>
> In the final analysis, the drug did not prove to be effective. The studies were flawed in their design and execution such that little definitive data were available; those data that could be interpreted suggested no difference between the Vitamin A drops and the placebo drops. The investigators' studies might well have been influenced by the promise of pecuniary gain.

Although not everyone would agree that pecuniary gain is a stronger biasing influence than recognition, the societal view is almost certainly one of expecting the desire for money to be more corrupting than the desire for fame. In the preceding case, the pecuniary aspects of the event caused it to become newsworthy not only for the scientific community (Booth 1988) but also for the general public (Chase 1989, Gosselin 1988).

The ophthalmology case also provides some insight into the borders between conflict of interest and fraud. As it turns out, some of the investigators sold portions of their stock for a tidy profit before it was generally known that the drug was ineffective and the stock plunged in price. Should one be able to prove that the investigators were willfully altering or withholding scientific data, the issue is no longer one of mere conflict of interest, but scientific fraud (Institute of Medicine 1989) and perhaps "insider trading." A lawsuit against the investigators has been filed by the investors/stockholders, charging deception (Levine 1990).

CONCLUSIONS

The preceding discussion, although quite superficial from the standpoint of the expert in basic and clinical study design, makes clear the importance of bias control. Not only must every effort be made in study design to minimize bias, but also investigators must be chosen who a priori have maximal reasons to be objective and minimal reasons to influence the study in a specific direction. We cannot eliminate the desire for recognition for the hard work of a scientific investigation. We can, however, exert some control on the investigators' pecuniary gain.

REFERENCES

Booth, W. 1988. Conflict of interest eyed at Harvard. *Science,* 242: 1497–9.

Chalmers, T. C. 1983a. The control of bias in clinical trials. *In Clinical Trials: Issues and Approaches.* New York: Marcel Dekker, 115.

Chalmers, T. C., et al. 1983b. Bias in treatment assignment in controlled clinical trials. *New England Journal of Medicine,* 309: 1358–61.

Chase, M. 1989. Bad chemistry: Mixing science, stocks raises question of bias in the testing of drugs. *Wall Street Journal,* 213(18): 1.

Committee on the Conduct of Science, National Academy of Sciences. 1989. *On Being a Scientist.* Washington, D.C.: National Academy Press.

Committee on Labor and Human Resources, United States Senate. 1991. Committee hearing. 101st Congress 2nd session.

Council on Scientific Affairs and Council on Ethical and Judicial Affairs. 1990. Conflict of interest in medical center, industry research relationships. *Journal of the American Medical Association,* 263(20): 2790–93.

Dudley, H. A. F. 1983. The controlled clinical trial and the advance of reliable knowledge: An outsider looks in. *British Medical Journal,* 287: 957–60.

Friedman, L. M., Furberg C. D., and DeMets, D. L. 1985. *Fundamentals of Clinical Trials.* Littleton, Massachusetts: PSG Publishing.

Gosselin, P. G. 1988. Flawed study helps doctors profit on drug. *Boston Globe,* 234(111): 1–2.

Healy, B., et al. 1989. Special report: Conflict-of-interest guidelines for a multicenter clinical trial of treatment after coronary-artery bypass-graft surgery. *New England Journal of Medicine,* 320: 949–51.

Institute of Medicine. 1989. IOM report of a study on the responsible conduct of research in the health sciences. *Clinical Research,* 37: 179–91.

Kneller, G. F. 1978. *Science as a Human Behavior.* New York: Columbia University Press.

Levine, J. 1990. Technology tales. *Johns Hopkins Magazine,* August, pp. 14–31.

Porter, R. J. 1988. *Recent Advances in Epilepsy.* Edinburgh, Scotland: Churchill Livingstone.

Weiss, T. 1989. Research that the U.S. government is paying for should not be tainted by any possibility of bias. *Chronicle of Higher Education.*

Woolgar, S. 1988. *Science: The Very Idea.* New York: Tavistock, Ellis Horwood.

10 • How to Control Conflict of Interest

Allan C. Shipp

Academic faculty members are engaged in a network of complex relationships as a natural outcome of their professional responsibilities. These include interactions with university co-workers, academic colleagues, and industrial and federal supporters of research. In addition, each faculty member has a unique matrix of personal obligations and interests that are equally diverse. The potential for conflicts among these various roles and responsibilities is ever-present.

Particular attention has been drawn recently to faculty activities at the interface of academia and industry. The growing commercial opportunity presented by new developments in biomedicine (particularly biotechnology) and the increasing significance of industrial funds in undergirding academic research have contributed to a climate in which faculty contacts with industry are expanding at an unprecedented rate. With that expansion has developed increasing concern among some policymakers that private interests (either personal or commercial) may be inappropriately influencing publicly funded research. Although a loss of objectivity or commitment is not an inevitable outcome of faculty contacts with the commercial sector, even the perception that such could occur gives cause for a reexamination of the various roles and obligations held by the investigator. Conflicting situations, whether perceived or real, inflict long-term damage on societal trust and support of research. More important, the bias that conflicting interests may interject has the potential to lead investigators to inappropriate research conclusions and ultimately to clinical practices or products that are ineffective or even dangerous.

The public policy question is, then, how to deal with the eventuality of conflicts of interest among biomedical researchers. Some have proposed that conflicts be eliminated and sources of conflict be precluded. Others would argue that the elimination of all conflicts is an unfeasible and undesirable goal. Many conflicts are not, in fact, of a pecuniary nature. It can be argued that there are personal, intangible rewards that can create conflicts with the scientist's search for truth that can never be eliminated, nor should they be. Kept in perspective, the quest for achievement, or for validation of one's ideas, serve to keep scientists motivated and pursuing new research directions. In addition, there are equally valid and necessary rewards in the research system that should not be stifled. For example, positive research results per se may contribute to opportunities for publication, promotion, tenure, grant renewals, and so forth. Again, such incentives keep the research system productive, and their elimination would discourage new entrants from pursuing a field already threatened with declining participation.

Therefore, if such incentives cannot and should not be eliminated, how do we ensure that they are indeed kept in perspective and do not cause deviation from objectivity in the design, interpretation, and publication of research activities—or other academic and professional decisions for that matter? Rather than eliminating incentives, the goal should be to create appropriate controls in the system to ensure the integrity of the scientific process and the validity of conclusions drawn from the research data. The key elements of such a system are disclosure and independent scrutiny of one's research.

One might question whether the data themselves should require validation through independent audit, but consideration of this issue requires some risk:benefit comparisons. As discussed in other chapters, clinical trials entail very significant potential risks to human health, some immediate and some long term. Before products are brought onto the market, there must be an extremely high degree of certainty that they are safe and efficacious. In light of these issues and the sheer expense and difficulty in replicating these trials, it is appropriate to scrutinize clinical trial protocols and data very closely. The U.S. Food and Drug Administration (FDA) has created a system in which such rigorous outside review occurs. On the other hand, for basic research that occurs at the lab bench, rather than at the clinical bedside, such intensive verification of raw data on a federal or institutional level would be extremely costly and time consuming and would accomplish little beyond what is now achieved by the normal process of peer review and replication.

EXTRAINSTITUTIONAL CONTROLS

Given these considerations, what mechanisms of control should be in place? The first controls that are considered herein are those developed outside the administrative procedures of the academic institution: self-control, peer review, and governmental requirements.

Self-control

The most fundamental means of control is, simply put, self-control. In the context of this discussion, honesty is assumed. A sociopath who is intent on deception and on defeating the system will probably succeed, at least to a limited extent, no matter what controls are in place. Such individuals must be dealt with through mechanisms designed to deal with deliberate and improper conduct. These mechanisms should be procedurally distinct from those to address inadvertent conflicts of interest or the possible introduction of unwanted bias. However, even honest scientists must be sensitive to the potential for conflicts of interest and must monitor their own behavior. For example, choices of research questions and protocols should be carefully evaluated and reevaluated in light of inadvertently satisfying interests not directly relevant to the science at hand. Self-elimination from potentially conflicting activities may be key to self-regulation as well. Bernadine Healy and other members of her research team at the Cleveland Clinic investigating post coronary-artery-bypass graft (CABG) surgery treatments, announced in 1989 the following voluntarily imposed self-restrictions:

> Investigators involved in the Post CABG study will not buy, sell, or hold stock or stock options in any of the companies providing or distributing medication under study . . . for the following periods: from the time the recruitment of patients of the trial begins until funding for the study in the investigator's unit ends and the results are made public; or from the time the recruitment of patients for the trial begins until the investigator's active and personal involvement in the study or the involvement of the institution conducting the study (or both) ends. (Healy et al. 1989)

The group similarly restricted themselves from consultancy positions in the companies involved, and it imposed annual reporting requirements concerning the participation of investigators in educational activities supported by the companies, the participation in other research projects supported by the companies, and uncompensated consulting to the companies on unrelated issues.

The ability of this team to remain objective in light of the afore-mentioned interests may have been one concern precipitating this move. Equally important, perhaps, was the question of public percep-tion and the apparent credibility of the team's research findings when such interests are held. This latter concern is important and should be kept in mind in the process of self-regulation.

Peer Review

Another key form of control relates to the peer review inherent in the scientific process. Integral to this form of control is the understand-ing that scientists make honest mistakes, and uncovering those mis-takes is a natural part of the scientific process. After the completion of the experiment, findings are conveyed to the scientific and general pub-lic through publication in the literature. Methodologies and conclusions are evaluated by journal editors, reviewers, and eventually the inter-ested readership. They are often tested, particularly in the case of the most significant or seminal research, through duplication of the re-search protocol. A dialogue is created among scientists, and many er-roneous or flawed experiments are identified as such in this way. For ground-breaking research, the attention of the media is often drawn, and the research becomes the focus of much public scrutiny. Invalid results are often quickly identified in such cases.

Peer review as an exclusive form of control is not ideal, however, because it may not result in the recognition of mistakes in the most arcane research and fails to address the notion of bias when it is most productive to do so—a priori. The discovery of a conflict of interest "after the fact," particularly in the case of a finding that has captured the public's attention, will serve to undermine the credibility and rep-utation not only of the scientist involved, but also of the scientific profession as a whole. Under these circumstances, questions of impro-priety, wasteful expenditures of public funds, and possible public harm arise, and the research community risks being viewed as unwilling or unable to deal with investigator conflicts. The public then demands greater federal controls, and the U.S. Congress and the federal agen-cies become involved.

Federal Requirements

The executive branch of the federal government has particular re-quirements for institutional controls and is interested in expanding its role. For biomedical research, which is the focus of this chapter, the most relevant and active agency is the Public Health Service (PHS). It is currently a PHS requirement that grantee institutions have conflict-of-interest policies in place. The 1990 PHS Grants Policy Statement says,

> Recipient organizations must establish safeguards to prevent employees, consultants, or members of governing bodies from using their positions for purposes that are, or give the appearance of being, motivated by a desire for private financial gain for themselves or others such as those with whom they have family business, or other ties. Therefore, each institution receiving financial support must have written policy guidelines on conflict of interest and the avoidance thereof. These guidelines should reflect State and local laws and must cover financial interests, gifts, gratuities and favors, nepotism, and other areas such as political participation and bribery. (Public Health Service, U.S. Department of Health and Human Services 1990)

The PHS statement adds that such policies must include provisions for implementation and sanctions for violations. In September 1989, two component agencies of the PHS, the National Institutes of Health (NIH) and the Alcohol, Drug Abuse and Mental Health Administration (ADAMHA), issued a controversial proposal to deal more explicitly with conflicts of interest (National Institutes of Health and Alcohol, Drug Abuse and Mental Health Administration 1989). This proposed "guideline" would have prohibited those directly involved in NIH- or ADAMHA-funded research or their immediate families from having personal equity holdings or options in "any company that would be affected by the outcome of the research." It also would have (1) forbidden the receipt of any honoraria, fees-for-service, or management position from research sponsors, (2) required disclosure of *all* financial interests and professional activities, and (3) placed severe restrictions on information sharing with relevant companies. PHS received more than 700 responses to that proposal, most of which were highly critical. As a consequence, on December 29, Health and Human Services Secretary Louis Sullivan retracted the proposal, stating, "While there is a crucial need to protect against possible abuses in the research system, it is also important that we not impose on our scientific community regulatory burdens which may be unnecessary or counterproductive." He asked NIH to redraft a proposal that would be "free of unnecessary burdens and disincentives." Sullivan also required that the next proposal follow a more formal rule-making process that would result in legally enforceable regulations rather than guidelines (Sullivan 1989). As of this writing, NIH and ADAMHA are in the process of developing a new regulatory proposal, spurred on in part by some U.S. Congressional representatives who are interested in seeing more done to control the effects that conflicts of interest may have on federally sponsored research.

INSTITUTIONAL CONTROLS

Clearly, if the research institutions themselves were viewed by policymakers as being more effective at controlling the biases that may be introduced by conflicts of interest, there would be less impetus for development of additional controls at the federal level. For reasons of proximity to faculty and their activities, it is, in fact, at the institutional level that controls are most effectively implemented. Such controls, in the form of policies and procedures for dealing with conflicts of interest, work in tandem with the mechanisms of control built into the scientific process. Institutional policies and procedures are generally focused on sources of conflict rather than elimination of bias. The scientific process, if functioning properly, should contain controls that promote unbiased observation, regardless of the sources of bias.

It behooves institutions to have effective policies and procedures in place. If functioning well, such policies and procedures can promote integrity, enhance the quality of research, protect human subjects, and safeguard research funds. Other than meeting federal requirements, policies and procedures must be developed in recognition of the unique circumstances each institution faces with regard to state laws, organizational structure, varying degrees and levels of involvement in industry, faculty activities, codes of conduct, and so forth. Understandably, there is no pat policy for dealing with these complex questions. Apart from these considerations, there are elements of policies that have no single "right" or "correct" approach, such as where to set thresholds for certain activities; these elements must be decided in accordance with the wisdom of relevant institutional officials, as discussed next.

Because consulting and collaboration with industry are perceived to play a significant role in creating sources of conflict, institutional policies and procedures must deal with these relationships. One source of conflict posed by these opportunities pertains to financial incentives for bias, and another concerns failure to live up to the primary duties attendant to one's position at the employing institution. Although this chapter is concerned with bias in research, conflicts related to distribution of effort—conflicts of commitment—are related and may be dealt with in the same policies as those concerning conflicts of interest. The question of conflicts of commitment, however, are discussed elsewhere in this book.

EXTERNAL GUIDANCE ON INSTITUTIONAL POLICY DEVELOPMENT

Early guidance on dealing with conflicts of interest was issued in 1964 jointly by the Council of the American Association of University Professors (AAUP) and the American Council on Education (ACE). Their statement, "On Preventing Conflicts of Interest in Government-Sponsored Research at Universities" (American Association of University Professors and the American Council on Education 1964), was intended to assist academic institutions in defining conflict situations and university responsibility to address conflicts. The document was limited in scope (two pages in length) and served principally in aiding institutions in conceptualizing the issue. Nonetheless, the AAUP-ACE piece served as the template for a large number of institutional policies developed after its publication.

In the next twenty years, very little institutional guidance on dealing with conflicts of interest was published. Then in 1983, with the help of a grant from the Pew Memorial Trust, the Association of American Universities (AAU) established the Clearinghouse on University-Industry Relations. This project was undertaken in response to a 1981 request from the Oversight Committee of the House Committee on Science and Technology to develop ethical guidelines to govern academic-industry collaboration. Rather than develop uniform guidelines, the AAU chose instead to establish a clearinghouse that would "provide all interested parties with information about the policies and practices governing the growing connections between universities and industry" (Association of American Universities 1985). Two reports emanated from this project; the first outlined elements of policies concerning conflict of interest and delays in publication, and the second report dealt with trends in technology transfer.

As concerns among policymakers heightened once again in the late 1980s over conflict of interest in research, a number of constituent groups began work on guiding their membership in policy development. Between late 1989 and 1990, the American Medical Association issued a number of white papers on various facets of the conflict-of-interest issue. One of these publications, published in the *Journal of the American Medical Association* (American Medical Association 1990), focused on clinical research activity and provided broad recommendations for professional societies and medical centers to follow in policy development.

In early 1990, a committee of the Association of Academic Health Centers (AHC) issued *Conflict of Interest in Academic Health Centers*

(Association of Academic Health Centers 1990), a piece that gives significant consideration to the large variety of academic-industry links that may present various forms of conflicts. The AHC document considers a number of different venues, including research, clinical activities, and education, and it outlines principles that should serve as the basis for guidelines in each setting.

During the same time, the Association of American Medical Colleges (AAMC) worked to provide its membership with explicit guidance in developing policies and procedures to deal with this issue. The outcome of that process was the *Guidelines for Dealing with Faculty Conflicts of Commitment and Conflicts of Interest in Research* (Association of American Medical Colleges 1990). As the title suggests, the AAMC report focuses exclusively on conflicts in the research setting. A major exercise in development of that document was the solicitation of policies from AAMC member institutions such that various elements of a comprehensive policy could be identified. The author of this chapter, serving as staff to this effort, reviewed these policies to compare how different institutions had dealt with various aspects of policy development.

In the course of reviewing policies for the AAMC effort, the basic components to a sound institutional policy became evident. These include

1. Explicit definition of conflict of interest, often illustrated with examples
2. Clearly defined scope of policy (e.g., affected individuals and institutions)
3. Effective procedural elements
   a. Timely disclosure of relevant information
   b. Thorough review of disclosed information
   c. Mechanism for management and/or resolution of conflict situations
4. Sanctions for policy violation

The rest of this chapter identifies options for each of these policy elements, with examples of how research institutions and the organizations they turn to for guidance have dealt with each. It should be kept in mind that almost all of the institutional policies cited herein were developed before the recent AHC and AAMC guidelines and all before any PHS regulation in this area. The current period of time is one of flux for conflict-of-interest policy development, and many institutions are revising policies to address ongoing concerns. Unfortunately, as of this writing, it is too early to assess the impact of the most recent guidelines on institutional policy development.

INSTITUTIONAL POLICIES AND PROCEDURES

Definition and Scope

The first step in dealing with conflicts of interest is to define those situations that ought to be of concern to the institution. Generally, institutional policies use the term *conflict of interest* to encompass a number of situations that compromise the credibility and public perception of the faculty member and other officers of the university. As the 1990 report of the AHC noted, "Like many important concepts, 'conflict of interest' is susceptible to many meanings . . . a useful discussion of conflicts of interest must begin with a definition that excludes conflicts that are trivial or unavoidable" (AHC Report 1990). The AHC report concluded that a workable definition is that "a potential or actual conflict of interest exists when legal obligations or widely recognized professional norms are likely to be compromised by a person's other interest, particularly if those interests are not disclosed" (AHC Report 1990).

In their 1964 joint statement, the ACE and the AAUP did not so much define conflicts as illustrate them with situations in which conflicts of interest might arise and give at least the appearance of favoring outside interests. Such situations include (1) undertaking research oriented to the needs of a private firm, (2) purchasing equipment or other materials from a firm in which a personal interest exists, (3) inappropriate transmission of the products of government-sponsored work, for personal gain, (4) inappropriate use of privileged information, (5) influencing negotiation of contracts related to government-sponsored research, and (6) acceptance of gratuities from firms with which the university conducts business on government-sponsored contracts.

In its 1990 guidance, the AAMC defined the term *conflicts of interest in research* as "situations in which financial or other personal considerations may compromise, or have the appearance of compromising, an investigator's professional judgment in conducting or reporting research" (AAMC 1990). Similarly, situations that may at the very least give the appearance of a conflict of interest are described in the AAMC document, to alert institutions to the kinds of activities that should, at the very least, require close scrutiny.

An important common thread in all these definitions is the question of dealing with even the appearance of a conflict—which is critical if questions of public confidence in research are to be addressed. Another common element found in many definitions, including those of the AHC and the AAMC, is the importance of distinguishing *conflicts of interest,* which most definitions relate to the injection of inappropriate bias, from *conflicts of commitment* (distribution of effort and time), and from outright fraud in research.

Most institutional policies employ definitions that are quite broad, encompassing more than simply research activities: "Typically, a conflict of interest may arise when a [faculty] member has the opportunity to influence the University's business, administrative, academic or other decisions in ways that could lead to personal gain or advantage of any kind" (Cornell University Medical College 1986). "In the conventional sense, conflict of interest refers to situations in which employees may have the opportunity to influence the University's business decisions in ways that could lead to personal gain or give advantage to associates of firms in which employees have an interest" (University of California 1984a).

Some policies, such as Cornell's, then address conflicts of interest in research and nonresearch activities collectively. Others, such as the University of California system, have developed a number of separate policies, some tailored specifically to research activities. The former approach recognizes that objectivity is key in any professional activity and that a given activity or interest may have implications beyond research. The latter approach, however, often creates a more explicit procedural link to institutional sponsored-research activities, facilitating disclosure and review. Either approach may be appropriate, provided gaps are not left in the scope of conflicts that ought to be addressed and the institutional procedures necessary to identify and manage conflicts on a regular basis.

Models

Most institutional policies employ one (or some combination) of three models for further defining and classifying conflicts of interest. The three prevalent models are

1. Prohibiting particular types of activities that pose conflicts
2. Classifying activities according to varying levels of scrutiny and control
3. Reviewing activities on a case-by-case basis, with no prohibitions or classifications a priori

Prohibition

Some institutions explicitly prohibit certain relationships or activities, either because they are viewed as unmanageable sources of bias or because the institution believes they would create unmitigable public concern over the potential for bias. Stanford states that "certain situations must be avoided since even full disclosure would not satisfy University or contractual requirements and approval of such actions could not be granted by the University" (Stanford University 1979).

Examples of such situations are provided in the policy and are very similar to the 1965 AAUP/ACE guidelines: unauthorized transmission of university-supported work products, materials, information, and so forth; use of privileged information for personal gain; negotiating contracts with a firm in which an individual has a significant relationship; and either accepting gratuities or special favors from private organizations with which the university conducts business or extending favors for influencing outside organizations. These types of prohibitions are relatively noncontroversial and would probably be excluded from acceptable faculty behavior by most institutions. Although many institutional conflict-of-interest policies address these activities (perhaps because of the influence of the AAUP/ACE document), such activity may be covered by other schools in separate institutional policies dealing with appropriate faculty conduct.

However, recent U.S. Congressional concerns have been raised regarding conflicts of interest related to the possibly biasing effects of financial or managerial interests in companies that sponsor research; several organizations have taken a stand on this issue. The AMA recommends prohibiting *financial transactions* that may relate to the research in question: "Once a clinical investigator becomes involved in a research project for a company or knows that he or she might become involved, the investigator, as an individual, cannot ethically buy or sell the company's stock until the involvement ends and the results of the research are published or otherwise disseminated to the public" (American Medical Association 1990).

However, a small number of academic institutions have taken this concern with equity interests a step further by prohibiting *ownership* of relevant financial interests altogether: "A faculty member, the faculty member's spouse and minor children may not own or control stock or stock options (equity, shares) in a company at any time while that company is also supporting his or her academic work through financial or in-kind means, including support of the academic work of supervised faculty, nonfaculty employees and students" (Johns Hopkins School of Medicine 1989).

Interestingly enough, such prohibitions often do not address entities that may have equally strong interests in the outcome of the research, such as those competing with either the sponsor of research or the manufacturer of the product under evaluation. In addition, prohibitions may be limited to the faculty member (though this is not the case in the preceding example) and may not include *potentially* relevant family members and associates. In fact, the greatest difficulty with this approach is in defining the prohibitions such that they address *all* situations, potentially of legitimate concern.

The decision as to whether some form of blanket prohibition on financial and/or managerial interests should be implemented is best made at the institutional level. Mandating such prohibitions as an element of a public-policy approach is questionably effective in eliminating bias and is rather controversial. As alluded to earlier, pat prohibitions cannot address all situations that are potentially of concern and, in that sense, fail to achieve in a defensible manner the public-policy objective of ensuring the integrity of research. Prohibiting all situations potentially of concern would require precluding possibly appropriate, or even desirable arrangements, as only some subset would prove to be legitimately of concern after review. More limited, locally imposed prohibitions, however, can be integrated into an overall framework of policies and procedures that will ensure appropriate management of these borderline cases.

Classification

The second model is employed by Harvard Medical School (Harvard University Faculty of Medicine 1990). Activities are evaluated for classification as either (1) relationships/activities of greatest concern—allowable only after approval and oversight (Category I), (2) relationships/activities normally permissible following disclosure and perhaps oversight (Category II), or (3) activities that are routinely allowable (Category III). The policy provides explicit examples of the types of activities that would fall under each heading. Harvard Medical School does not prohibit a priori any particular relationship but focuses instead on case-by-case examination. A particularly useful aspect of the classification model is that it offers clarity concerning what constitutes appropriate and potentially inappropriate faculty behavior. In this way, many conflict situations may be avoided—a preferable situation than having to resolve conflicting arrangements once they are in place. In addition, the examples of situations, graded by the level of concern they prompt, provide faculty with a scale against which to gauge other, potentially relevant activities.

Case by Case

Some institutions deal with possible conflicts of interest on a case-by-case basis. Institutions that adopt this approach may do so quite legitimately, finding that (a) prohibitions cast either too broad or too incomplete a net, and (b) classification systems are too structured for the extremely variable situations they may face. This approach, however, is more administratively complex and requires great emphasis on education, disclosure, and conflict management. The importance of sensitizing faculty to potentially problematic situations is heightened by this approach because faculty will lack explicit prohibitions or classification schemes for prompting disclosures. Because specific activities for review have not been defined at the outset, a very broad range of activities must be disclosed to capture all potentially problematic situations. Finally, the lack of explicit outcomes attached to particular situations (such as outright prohibition) means that university administration must give more thought to how conflicting situations will be managed. It is important to note that inconsistent administration of policy is one possible risk associated with completely ad hoc management of conflict situations. Earlier institutional decisions on similar situations must be considered in conflict review, and differences in outcome must be carefully justified.

The Process of Disclosure

There is wide variation in how disclosure issues are handled procedurally among institutions, though once again, there are prevalent models both in terms of timing and process.

Disclosures are generally submitted either annually, on an ad hoc basis, or both. In many policies, a measure of responsibility is placed on the faculty member to recognize potentially conflicting situations: "The responsibility in the first instance for determining whether an outside activity presents a conflict of interest or commitment rests with the faculty member concerned. If there is any reasonable doubt as to whether an outside activity may constitute such a conflict, the faculty member must consult his or her dean" (New York University [NYU] 1984).

It should be noted that in addition to placing a measure of responsibility upon the faculty member, NYU does have a mechanism for university-initiated disclosure, through a form submitted annually in which compensated professional activity, management and directorial relationships, and significant financial interests are to be reported. This is important, for complete reliance on faculty members to identify their own conflicts is a risky approach. Faculty members cannot be entirely objective about their own activities and, thus, independent evaluation, through a university-initiated mechanism of disclosure is key.

One circumstance that should precipitate disclosure is the initiation of a sponsored research proposal. One school (University of California, Los Angeles 1986) states that a disclosure form must be filed by faculty:

1. When a proposal for a contract or grant (to support research) of $250 or more from a non-governmental entity is submitted, or, before final acceptance of a gift from a non-governmental entity that is earmarked by the donor for a specific research project or a specific principal investigator, provided the amount of the gift, or the aggregate over a 12-month period from the same donor, is $250 or more;
2. When contract or grant funding is renewed; and
3. Within 90 days after expiration of a contract or grant; or, in the case of a gift, after funds have been completely expended

In addition to these ad hoc disclosures, annual reporting of relevant staff activities is wise, to capture any changes in faculty status that faculty otherwise might neglect to report in a timely fashion.

Procedurally, disclosure review varies by institution and within institutions according to what event may have precipitated disclosure. One paradigm of review occurs in *bottom-up fashion,* following upward through the lines of authority within the university structure. If disclosure is relevant to a sponsored research proposal, an associate dean for research, sponsored projects officer, or other equivalent official might serve in the first level of review, as well. The AAMC recommends in its guidelines that disclosure first occur at the level of the department chair or primary supervisor. Subsequent reviews would occur at the level of the dean and eventually by a standing committee when additional review and conflict resolution is required. Having the primary supervisor as the first line of review carries the risk that the reviewer will be too close to the situation to view it objectively. On the other hand, familiarity with the individual and the science involved certainly has advantages when it comes to making an informed evaluation. In addition, faculty should have a mechanism at their disposal for informal consultations on situations that have created uncertainty for them.

Many policies provide for a committee to review potential instances of conflict of interest. Usually the committee is designated as a standing committee. Some committees are used in a mostly advisory role, to provide objective guidance when lower levels of review have failed to resolve whether a conflict exists: "To provide advice and if necessary make determinations [in situations where conflicts are uncertain], there is established a University Committee on Institutional Responsibility. That Committee shall consist of a Chairperson and six members, all of whom shall be tenured members of the faculty, and who shall be appointed for staggered three-year terms by the Chancellor after consultation with the Faculty Council" (New York University 1984).

In other instances, the committee's work begins when the disclosure process reveals an actual conflict: "When disclosure indicates that a financial interest exists, an independent substantive review of the disclosure statement and the research project must take place prior to acceptance of the contract, grant, or gift" (University of California 1984b).

Often, the committee depends on other university staff in evaluating possible conflicts of interest. Expertise may be solicited, as necessary, from the institution's offices of legal counsel, research administration, government relations, and technology transfer. The university, therefore, must be committed to supporting committee activities. In that vein, one policy reads,

> Chancellors, Laboratory Directors, and the Vice President . . . must provide the committees with appropriate administrative support, assure that technical advice on conflict of interest matters is provided, and assure that appropriate documents related to this policy are available to the public, as required by law.
>
> The Senior Vice President—Academic Affairs has responsibility for assuring compliance with applicable State law, this policy, and related University policies. He is responsible for developing and issuing implementing guidelines for this policy. He serves as the liaison on these matters with the Fair Political Practices Commission and with the campuses, Laboratories, and the Vice President—Agriculture and Natural Resources. He consults with the Senior Vice President—Administration when financial reporting by principal investigators affect the Senior Vice President. (University of California System 1984b)

Content of Disclosure

Disclosure requirements vary not only by process but also by content. Disclosure forms, for example, typically follow two models. One model is to require faculty to fill out a university-initiated form that results in disclosure of a broad range of potentially relevant outside activities (the elements of which are described in greater detail later herein), such that institutional officials may identify "red flags," or interests that at least raise concerns related to the appearance of conflicts of interest. The University of Illinois at Champaign-Urbana takes such an approach (University of Illinois, Champaign-Urbana 1989). Excessive time spent on nonuniversity activities and interests in firms relevant to university business or research are examples of reported activities that would trigger further investigation by university officials to determine whether a conflict exists. The other model is to rely on the faculty member to understand and recognize potentially conflicting situations, aided by text in the policy, which explains prohibited situations or situations requiring some level of review. Johns Hopkins University (JHU) Medical School, for example, calls for a faculty-initiated written report when certain potentially problematic conditions pertain (e.g., outside commitments in excess of twenty-six days per year, when the name of the institution might be used by another party, when a proposed agreement involves the use of facilities or resources belonging to JHU, and so forth) (Johns Hopkins 1989).

The former model (university-initiated forms) generally results in casting a very broad net to identify what often is a very small number of problem situations. The latter model (faculty-initiated) will produce less irrelevant information but requires greater reliance on faculty members to be vigilant and objective about their own activities.

The range of activities to be disclosed varies considerably from institution to institution. Disclosure requirements tend to be more stringent for the state (public) institutions, due to mandatory compliance with statutes applicable to state employees. For both public and private institutions, when disclosure is addressed, the following financial and managerial activities may be targeted:

1. *Equity Holdings*—Disclosure requirements for equity holdings vary among institutions, in terms of the amount and nature of the investments that trigger disclosure. Policies typically address only interests in companies that have some ongoing relationship to the university (research sponsor, contractor, supplier, etc.) rather than asking for full disclosure of all personal investments. This is probably justified both on a cost:benefit basis and on a right-to-privacy basis. Reporting thresholds may be set as either a percentage interest in the firm (e.g., 5 percent or 10 percent ownership of a company) or as a dollar limit (e.g., $10,000 for all investments, or $1,000 for the sponsor of research). Both approaches have their limitations. Thresholds based on a percentage interest of a company fails to recognize the potential significance of that investment relative to the personal worth of the faculty member. On the other hand, employing dollar limitations instead is inherently arbitrary.

2. *Outside Professional Positions*—A sound policy should require disclosure of all outside professional activities involving salary. These, of course, would include consulting arrangements, but other activities are of concern as well, including managerial and board positions.

3. *Outside Professional Income*—Disclosures of outside income are potentially relevant. Such disclosure may involve thresholds. One

medical school asks for disclosure of income greater than $250 from the sponsor; another asks for disclosure of all income in excess of $10,000 annually. Some ask for reports of any nonuniversity income-producing activity. Although thresholds may be useful in screening out inconsequential interests, they are inherently arbitrary and are difficult to defend.

4. *Gifts*—Frequently, gifts are overlooked or are perhaps assumed to be encompassed by the term *outside income*. Of course, gifts are not always monetary in nature and may be excluded by such assumptions. Some institutions prohibit gifts from agencies dealing with the institutions; others simply discourage their receipt; still others set limits on the value of those gifts ($50 and $100 are both caps used in some policies). For public institutions, state statutes frequently apply, and faculty are subject to the same restrictions or prohibitions as other state employees.

5. *Honoraria*—This may be disclosed separately or as an element of outside professional income.

6. *Loans*—A number of policies ask for disclosure of loans made by either research sponsors or companies dealing with the medical school or university. Some set acceptable limits (e.g., $250), and others require disclosure of any loan amount.

An area that many policies overlook is the potential for conflicts among outside interests. The type of situation in which this might arise is best illustrated in the following text:

> Faculty members are often called upon to act as consultants in the professions, to advise on the conduct of research, or to give expert testimony before a court of law. Such experts may find themselves in the employ of several clients whose interests are competitive in nature. All types of conflicts to which attention was called in the foregoing section are potentially present here as well. For example, a faculty member may well be consulted with regard to equipment needed for a laboratory installation to be operated by a private concern, and may thus have to choose among suppliers of equipment in some of whom he or she has a substantial interest.
>
> The university as an institution can do little to "police" such conflicts, but can serve as a counsel and advice in these matters. (Vanderbilt University 1990–1)

Resolutions and Sanctions

Institutional policies are probably the least explicit when it comes to the means for resolving possible conflicts. This does not necessarily reflect a lack of commitment to the policy but more likely results from the difficulty in defining beforehand the means to address an extremely complex set of potential relationships.

To guide its institutions, the AAMC suggests that after appropriate evaluation, most situations will be found to be

- Unacceptable and thus prohibited, or
- Permitted with the implementation of one or more committee recommendations to preclude unreasonable levels of bias or inappropriate activities, or
- Permitted as is because the disclosed personal information does not represent a possible source of unreasonable bias or an inappropriate activity. (AAMC 1990)

Options described by the AAMC for resolving permissible, but potentially problematic situations include:

- Public disclosure of all relevant information,
- Reformulation of the research workplan,
- Close monitoring of the research project,
- Divestiture of relevant personal interests,
- Termination or reduction of involvement in the relevant research project,
- Termination of inappropriate student involvement in projects, and
- Severance of outside relationships that pose conflicts. (AAMC 1990)

When deliberate violation of institutional policies occurs, simply developing remedies to eliminate conflicts may no longer suffice, and sanctions should apply. These may be found within conflict-of-interest policies, or, as pertains, in other policies related to scientific misconduct or other standards of faculty conduct. For example, one university conflict-of-interest policy pertaining to all activities, not just research, reads

> The initiative and responsibility for reporting known conflicts of interest rests upon the individual and failure to make timely reports of significant known conflicts may be subject to disciplinary action. . . . Dismissal of faculty may be invoked only in cases where the conflict of interest is of such severity as to constitute "proven misconduct" sufficient to warrant termination of academic appointment for cause. In addition, failure to disclose a known conflict of interest may make the organization that is the subject of the conflict of interest ineligible to do business with the University. (University of Louisville 1983)

Another institution stated,

The Faculty of Medicine expects its members to comply fully and promptly with the policy, including the requirements of disclosure. Instances of deliberate breach of policy, including failure to file or knowingly filing an incomplete, erroneous, or misleading disclosure form, violations of the guidelines, or failure to comply with prescribed monitoring procedures, will be adjudicated in accordance with applicable disciplinary policies and procedures of the Faculty of Medicine and of the affiliated hospitals. Possible sanctions will include the following:

1. Formal admonition;
2. The inclusion in the Faculty Member's file of a letter from the Office of the Dean indicating that the individual's good standing as a member of the Faculty has been called into question;
3. Ineligibility of the Faculty Member to apply for grants, to seek Institutional Review Board (IRB) approval, or to supervise graduate students;
4. Nonrenewal of appointment;
5. Dismissal from the Faculty of Medicine. (Harvard University Faculty of Medicine 1990)

CONCLUSION

As discussed earlier, the goal in managing conflicts of interest is not to eliminate all sources of conflicts of interest, an approach that clearly would be detrimental to research efforts locally and nationally, but instead to control the injection of inappropriate bias into research and other professional activities. This goal is worth pursuing, for such bias undermines both research credibility and the scientific process as a whole. In addition, faulty research conclusions may lead to products or practices that pose unacceptable threats to human health.

There is no single and universally applicable standard or formula for dealing with conflicts of interest. The heterogeneity of academic institutions and their partnerships and local requirements necessitate an institution-by-institution approach. This is not to say that institutions or their researchers should be without responsibility in this area. Indeed, both groups have a social and often a legal duty to ensure the integrity of *all* professional activities for which they are responsible.

In research, scientific investigators must exert some level of self-control. For example, they must be vigilant over their own biases, whether they stem from potential financial gain or merely from the desire to see their own ideas validated. In that vein, researchers must design carefully controlled experiments and seek challenges to their ideas from colleagues. Researchers must also be attentive to all other activities that relate or that might be perceived as relating to their research. Any that might detract from the credibility of research findings should either be discontinued before the research is undertaken or fully disclosed to all parties that have an interest in the research.

It would be unreasonable and unwise to depend entirely on the ability of researchers to identify, disclose, and manage all of their own potential conflicts of interest. The vast majority of researchers, and all people for that matter, are honest and will "do the right thing," provided they know what the "right thing" is. Distinguishing between questionable and acceptable practices is not always easy and often requires outside consultation and guidance. Thus, institutions have a weighty responsibility to aid researchers in monitoring and controlling their own activities. Elements of this institutional responsibility include the establishment of policies that delineate—insofar as possible—permissible and nonpermissible activities, mechanisms for timely disclosure of relevant faculty activities, and procedures for policy implementation and enforcement.

An interesting question is whether institutions themselves are sufficiently detached from the activities of their own investigators to identify and manage conflicts appropriately. Some policymakers have argued for stricter extrainstitutional controls, and proposals have been percolating for several years. In somewhat analogous fashion, extrainstitutional guidance and/or regulation was resisted but eventually accepted in the areas of animal welfare, human subjects, and—most recently—scientific misconduct. The need for federal regulations to govern conflicts of interest is still being hotly debated, and although it seems likely that such regulation will occur, the exact shape it will take is still unknown. Whatever the product of these extrainstitutional efforts, it must recognize the complexity of this issue and the need for institutional flexibility.

REFERENCES

American Association of University Professors and the American Council on Education. 1964. *On Preventing Conflicts of Interest in Government-Sponsored Research at Universities*. Washington, D.C.
American Medical Association. 1990. Report of the Council on Scientific Af-

fairs and the Council on Ethical and Judicial Affairs: Conflict of interest—Medical center-industry research relationships. *Journal of the American Medical Association,* 263(20): 2790–3.

Association of Academic Health Centers. 1990. *Conflicts of Interest in Academic Health Centers: A Report by the AHC Task Force on Science Policy.* Washington, D.C.

Association of American Medical Colleges. 1990. *Guidelines for Dealing with Faculty Conflicts of Commitment and Conflicts of Interest in Research,* Adopted by the AAMC Executive Council February 22, 1990. Washington, D.C.: AAMC Ad Hoc Committee on Misconduct and Conflict of Interest in Research.

Association of American Universities. 1985. *University Policies on Conflict of Interest and Delay of Publication: Report of the Clearinghouse on University-Industry Relations.* Washington, D.C.

Cornell University Medical College. 1986. *Cornell University Conflicts Policy for Cornell University Medical College and the Graduate School of Medical Sciences.* New York, New York.

Harvard University Faculty of Medicine. 1990. *Policy on Conflict of Interest and Commitment.* Boston, Massachusetts.

Healy, B. M., et al. 1989. Special report: Conflict-of-interest guidelines for a multicenter clinical trial of treatment after coronary-artery bypass-graft surgery. *New England Journal of Medicine,* 320(14): 951.

Johns Hopkins University School of Medicine. 1989. *Policy on Conflict of Commitment and Conflict of Interest.* Baltimore, Maryland.

National Institutes of Health and the Alcohol, Drug Abuse and Mental Health Administration. 1989. Request for comment on proposed guidelines for policies on conflict of interest. *NIH Guide for Grants and Contracts,* 18(32):

New York University. 1984. *Statement of Policy on Faculty Responsibility to the University* (December 10), p. 115-B.

Public Health Service, U.S. Department of Health and Human Services. 1990. *PHS Grant Policy Statement* (DHHS Publication No. 2, OASH, 90-50,000—rev. October 1); Section 8. Rockville, Maryland p. 17.

Stanford University. 1979. *Administrative Guide Memo 15.2.* Palo Alto, California.

Sullivan, L. 1989. *Statement by Health and Human Services Secretary Louis Sullivan on the NIH/ADAMHA Proposed Guidelines for Policies on Conflict of Interest.* Washington, D.C.

University of California, Los Angeles. 1986. *Disclosing Financial Interest in Private Sponsors of Research.* (UCLA Standard Procedure No. 921). Los Angeles, California.

University of California. 1984a. *Guidelines for Disclosure and Review of Principal Investigator's Financial Interest in Private Sponsors of Research.* Berkeley, California.

University of California. 1984b. *University Policy on Disclosure of Financial Interest in Private Sponsors of Research.* Berkeley, California.

University of Illinois, Champaign-Urbana. 1989. *Report of Non-University Activities*. Champaign-Urbana, Illinois.

University of Louisville. 1983. *Conflict of Interest Policy: Proposed Guidelines*. Louisville, Kentucky.

Vanderbilt University. 1990–1. *Faculty Manual*. Nashville, Tennessee.

PART IV

Industry and Government Views of Biomedical Collaboration

11 • The Research Needs of Industry: Working with Academia and with the Federal Government

Theodore Cooper and Mark Novitch

Collaboration in research between industry and academia or government is viewed by some as a new paradigm for research funding in the United States. In fact, what we have seen since the early 1980s is a return to a pattern of intimate relationships that existed between the two groups before World War II and the rapid growth of the National Institutes of Health (NIH) in the 1950s and 1960s. The funding of biomedical research has changed only to the extent that the technological base of biomedical research has changed and costs have increased—high costs now exist throughout the entire health care enterprise, from basic research to delivery of services.

As we explain in this chapter, there are many reasons other than monetary ones for collaboration between the pharmaceutical industry and academic medical centers. However, monetary concerns are now a major factor because the costs of both medical education and drug development are escalating rapidly.

In this chapter, we concentrate on collaborations between the pharmaceutical industry and academic medical centers. The basic principles and concerns set forth here apply, with some modifications, to collaboration with departments within universities and direct collaboration with the federal government (such as joint development of anticancer agents with the National Cancer Institute).

If one accepts that corporate funding has an appropriate and possibly even vital place inside academic medical centers, then the following basic principles should apply:

1. There is a long tradition of interaction between the pharmaceutical industry and research physicians, particularly in the United States, and this interaction has proven to be mutually beneficial.
2. Research is an integral element of an overall national health policy, which is influenced by a dynamic of costs, societal expectations, and technology.
3. In drug development, the time between discovery and initial application is decreasing, and pharmaceutical companies have a vital interest in leveraging that shortened time frame in order to create competitive advantages. As the time for development shrinks, it has become harder to distinguish basic from applied research. The blurring of this distinction is also of vital interest to patients and patient-advocacy groups.
4. There is nothing inherently corrupting about the presence of industrial funding in academic medical centers because all research funding has economic components and determinants.
5. Regulatory rules and requirements, not industry's profit-making orientation, are the major hindrance to academic-industry undertakings.
6. Technology transfer has greatly improved since the early 1980s and thus has mitigated many of the earlier concerns about patents, trade secrets, and delays in publishing research findings.
7. Collaborative agreements should not be rigidly uniform. Each should be individually tailored to achieve valid clinical ends, mutually agreeable financial results, and legally acceptable consequences. The concepts of "enlightened self-interest" and "the public interest" should guide all such collaborations.
8. The pattern of collaboration between industry and academia or government will only strengthen in the coming years. The course of public policy on health will be a major factor in determining the extent and fruitfulness of such collaborations.

HISTORICAL TRADITION OF INTERACTION BETWEEN THE PHARMACEUTICAL INDUSTRY AND RESEARCH PHYSICIANS

The story of the pharmaceutical industry in the United States is, in fact, largely written by physicians who were dissatisfied with the status quo in medicine (Mahoney 1959). The European industry had different origins because it grew out of the chemical and dye manufacturing industries. Japanese pharmaceutical companies developed similarly to those in Europe, although unlike most European companies, most Japanese companies now belong to huge conglomerates.

In the United States, Wallace Abbott—the founder of Abbott Laboratories—was intrigued by the possibility of precipitating the active principle of botanical drugs. He set up a rudimentary laboratory to make what he termed "dosimetric granules," which would be more uniform, pleasant, and palatable than the fluid extracts then in use.

Another example of the interaction between research physicians and the pharmaceutical industry is the story of Edward Squibb, founder of the company that is now part of Bristol-Myers Squibb Co. Squibb was a U.S. Navy doctor who was appalled at the contamination and deliberate adulteration of anesthetic ether and other drugs sold to the military. Squibb started a manufacturing laboratory at the Brooklyn Naval Hospital, where he invented, among other things, the process for producing pure, uniform anesthetic ether, a process that is still in use today. Squibb was also an important driving force in establishing the U.S. Pharmacopeia.

W. E. Upjohn, who founded our company in 1886, was troubled by the way medicines did not dissolve in patients' bodies—an early problem in bioavailability. To meet it, he developed a rapidly disintegrating pill, which he called a "friable pill," and built a business around it.

It took more than fifty years for most of the U.S. pharmaceutical companies to build up internal research and development (R&D) capabilities, which meant that working with academic researchers and physicians was a necessity. The products of this early collaboration—insulin, antibiotics (especially penicillin), and extracts for cardiovascular indications—are legend.

Today, the relationship extends beyond collaborative research agreements to consultancies, fellowships, and cross training. It is important to remember that direct research contracts and industry-funded research centers are only one part of a large network of interactions between industry and academic medical centers. No modern pharmaceutical company, given today's intense competitive dynamics, can exist without a strong clinical focus in its research program. Academic medical centers are a vital source of that focus.

Of course, sometimes, companies obtain a stronger clinical focus by hiring research physicians directly out of academic medical centers. A classic example involves P. Roy Vagelos, who was at the Washington University School of Medicine from 1966 until he joined Merck & Co in 1975. By 1986, Vagelos had become chair, president, and chief executive officer of that company.

More and more, we see similar situations, such as that involving Upjohn Laboratories, our corporate R&D operation. Jerry Mitchell, who as recently as 1988 was an academic collaborator with Upjohn at the Baylor College of Medicine, is now president of Upjohn Laboratories. In that sense, Upjohn and all other research-based companies have a vested interest in the health of all academic medical centers. This vested interest has always been there; it is not a recent phenomenon.

RESEARCH AS AN INTEGRAL ELEMENT OF NATIONAL HEALTH POLICY

No matter where research takes place or under what conditions it is conducted, it exists in a larger context shaped by a number of interactive and sometimes competing forces within health policy. Currently, we are in a phase where costs, societal expectations, and technology compete equally for attention in policy circles (Cooper 1990). Because health policy in this country is largely driven by economic considerations, the cost dimension receives the most attention. However, that does not mean that the flow of technology has ebbed or that society's expectations of the pharmaceutical industry are diminishing; the opposite is true. Technology continues to evolve at breathtaking speed. The closer we get to developing treatments for life-threatening or previously untreatable diseases and injuries, the more quickly society wants them.

All this means that pharmaceutical companies need to operate on as broad a front as possible to select the opportunities that best fit their capabilities and to develop those opportunities as rapidly as possible. Because the research enterprise is so diverse, and because it extends around the world, the research-based pharmaceutical companies must establish interfaces with basic and clinical research in a number of different ways and places.

The research base on which we operate is a triad of industry, academia, and government. No one portion of the triad can exist without the other. For instance, industry needs the NIH as much as any individual investigator does. Conversely, government and academic researchers need industry not only as a source of funding, but also as a source of development capability that leads to tangible and useful tools in health care.

The triad thus provides both symbiosis and synergy. The net effect is that biomedical research programs benefit from critical mass, economies of scale, and fresh perspectives in a way that maximizes the return on investment of research dollars. It does not matter from the public's point of view whether those dollars were originally invested in the public or the private sector, or a combination of the two. The public wants what everyone in the triad ultimately wants—improved patient care and comfort.

What industry needs from academic medical centers is not some short-term advantage. Our needs are long range: patients, prestige, patents, publications, and personnel. These so-called five Ps, in combination with the sixth P of profit, remain crucial to the vitality of every pharmaceutical company (Cooper 1988). These elements will be even more important as cost-containment measures impinge on the revenue stream, and as technological sophistication and increasing regulatory requirements drive up the cost of drug development.

RAPID INCREASES IN DISCOVERY-TO-DEVELOPMENT TIME

In 1985, *Science* addressed this issue as follows:

Innovation cannot occur without basic research as input, and basic research that does not lead to technological innovation in the form of marketable products and processes does little to better our quality of life. Too much emphasis has been placed on the dichotomy between the "pure," basic research done at universities and the applied research considered the province of industry. Rapid growth in scientific advancement has blurred the line separating the two. Increased interaction between universities and industry is inevitable as the federal government contributes an ever smaller portion of the research dollar; such relationships may prove to be the best way to serve the needs of all involved, including the public. (Varrin 1985)

It is important to note here that we are discussing initial applications of a discovery. In the development of a new pharmaceutical, the road to an Investigational New Drug (IND) application to a New Drug Application to an approved NDA is a long and risky one. However, the stronger the drug and product candidates the industry sends down the road, the more likely it is that an innovative and market-leading product will emerge.

The experience of the biotechnology industry in the 1980s offers an instructive example of how the issues surrounding research change rapidly. In one decade, we went from the concerns expressed at the Asilomar Conference in the 1970s to realistic questions about whether we even need the NIH guidelines on recombinant deoxyribonucleic acid (rDNA) research. Our point here is that what may seem like deep or even intractable issues in science have a way of diminishing over time as other, more fundamental, social issues change. It is our contention that this is precisely what is happening with academic-industry collaborations in research.

What has come to be called "biotechnology" is also driving research toward discovering the etiology of disorders, not just their palliation, as a consequence of the compression of the period between discovery and application. If one has discovered the role of a regulatory protein, for instance, and is able to clone the gene that expresses it, then one is far closer to a therapeutic agent than is someone who is screening thousands of compounds derived from organic chemistry. You are suddenly much closer to practical problems, such as how to deliver a large protein to a target organ or cell system. In other words, the aspects of clinical application of a discovery appear almost immediately after the discovery itself. This time-compression phenomenon would be bringing academic and industrial researchers closer together even if there were no such thing as federal budget deficits or periodic recessions (Schneiderman 1988).

While time compression creates more opportunities for a breakthrough therapy, it also creates competitive pressures. Shrinking patent life means that a marketed therapy needs to recover development costs and generate high earnings as fast as possible. The very successes of modern drug development also create competitive pressures. If one is designing a drug to block a specific receptor, for instance, it is easy for a competitor to take a slightly different approach to the same technology. The example provided by ranitidine as a competitor to cimetidine is a good one.

As we pointed out, only a highly flexible corporate research program can adapt in this new environment. Also, even as discovery and application are brought closer together, even as pharmaceutical companies begin to shorten development times, a number of basic problems are still slowing progress and can only be met by full cooperation in all sectors of the research triad. Some examples are the human genome (mapping and sequencing), protein structure, and folding; immune system modulation and the etiology of autoimmune diseases; brain chemistry and the blood-brain barrier, viral disease intervention (not just AIDS); and delivery of large proteins into the body. In this sense, the field on which academic medical centers, government, and industry will be playing in the future is extremely broad.

ECONOMIC NATURE OF RESEARCH FUNDING

Societal expectations—and demands—can and will interfere with the best-designed peer-review system and cause the most research dollars to follow the most au courant grant applications. The disease-of-the-month syndrome is one example of how grant applications follow priorities that are set through mechanisms other than pure science.

NIH grants themselves have important economic consequences for those holding and keeping them (Brody 1990). In fact, much of the supplementary income generated by the faculty of academic medical centers is achieved as much by virtue of holding a particular NIH grant as it is by holding a particular faculty position or having a particular research contract with a pharmaceutical company. In addition, there is pressure to enroll patients under NIH grants, which is another potential compromise in clinical research (Brody 1990).

This is not to say that conflict of interest (COI) is not a serious issue—it is. However, as is discussed at length elsewhere in this book, there are numerous examples and guidelines to follow in creating COI policies. Industry is engaging in self-defeating behavior if it encourages COI or any other abrogation of the research/clinical trials-marketing continuum.

Fraud is not the concern. Fraud is the act of desperate people. The point is that all parties must carefully structure collaborations so that unintended mistakes and misunderstandings are minimized.

REGULATIONS AS A MAJOR HINDRANCE TO ACADEMIC-INDUSTRY ENDEAVORS

This is particularly true in the case of the U.S. Food and Drug Administration (FDA), which in turn often serves as a model for regulatory systems elsewhere in the world. To the extent that FDA remains an underfunded, understaffed agency, we can expect little change in the agency's contribution to therapeutic innovation any time soon. The shrinking technical and scientific resources available to the FDA and their effect on academic-industry collaborations exemplify how a shortfall in one area of the research triad can have profound effects on other areas.

The need to fulfill regulatory requirements is more likely to conflict with the fundamental drives of clinical research at the protocol-design stage and less so in the implementation of a trial (Brody 1990). Surrogate endpoints and the trigger points for cutting a trial short are the main potential conflicts, which is why thoughtful and open negotiation is needed at the design stage.

Academic medical centers and industry should work in tandem with FDA management to develop more realistic sets of requirements and standards in the areas of active controls and large, community-based trials. This is particularly true in areas such as mental illness, acquired immunodeficiency syndrome (AIDS), cancer, and trauma.

We can expect to see more and more breakthrough products such as zidovudine (AZT) entering the clinical trials system in the future. Industry sponsors and their collaborators must be careful to ensure that research programs balance the needs of desperately ill patients with the scientific and medical integrity of the clinical trials process. The far-reaching effects of AIDS patient-advocacy groups prefigure future public pressures on clinical trials at large. We can expect, therefore, that the future of academic-industry collaborations will be related more and more to the process of developing therapies for previously untreatable diseases and to the attendant regulatory issues of expedited review, parallel track development, and treatment INDs.

CUSTOMIZATION OF COLLABORATIVE AGREEMENTS

Though collaborative agreements should be tailored for each collaboration, they should not evolve in an informal fashion. Each case is special and requires a special design. One would expect a different arrangement with a faculty member in the microbiology department at the University of Wisconsin than one would with a clinical investigator at the Harvard Medical School, for instance, because the primary missions of the individuals and their respective institutions are different.

The report of the Twentieth Century Fund Task Force on the Commercialization of Scientific Research put the matter this way: "In general, universities must learn to define their interests in working with corporations and then see to it that those interests are achieved. The Task Force believes that university-industry relations are more likely to work effectively when they are designed than when they evolve in an ad hoc fashion" (Sproull 1984).

Rational design of collaborative agreements means making sure that all financial details are spelled out and agreed upon and that the legal ramifications are dealt with before an agreement is executed and research actually begins. Neither side should do any of this in an attempt to give short shrift to the other. "Enlightened self-interest in the public interest" can be defined as pursuing individual goals within a matrix of integrity, ethics, and responsibility. It creates a win-win situation that benefits the public as well as the collaborating parties.

The key point is that within universities or academic medical centers, the question should always be, "What does this project hope to accomplish? Does it have real scientific or medical value?" Too often, everyone in the research enterprise gets lost in the details and loses sight of the ultimate goal, which is improved patient care. If partners in research agreements work backward from the macrocosm of patient care, they are less likely to trip over the microcosmic aspects of executing protocols, paying royalties, or disagreeing over where patent rights should reside.

Industrial partners also should remember that they often are purchasing at little or no cost access to the infrastructure of a research institution that has been built up, often with public funds, over a long period of time. Intangible assets should be accounted for in all agreements (Pinter 1990). Conversely, industry needs better direction from industrial leaders and medical school administrators on the proper use of clinical investigators in Phase IV activities and postmarketing promotions (Brody 1990). Industry cannot afford a perception on the part of the public that it is co-opting, in any way, the prominent scientists and physicians who are looked upon as leaders in the therapeutic areas of interest to industry sponsors.

IMPROVEMENTS IN TECHNOLOGY TRANSFER

The Technology Transfer Act and its sequelae have created a governmental template for moving projects from the discovery stage to the application stage. In addition, we now see many more internal structures in academic institutions, such as BCM Technologies at the Baylor College of Medicine, which act as arms-length transfer agents to maximize the return on collaborative research to the parent institution.

Many of these improvements in technology transfer have arisen out of competitiveness concerns. This is another example of how academic-industry collaborations can be part of larger public policy issues, in this case trade policy and governmental attitudes toward the competitiveness of U.S. industry.

It was widely thought in the early 1980s that the concerns of industrial partners regarding patents would interfere with the publication interests of academic collaborators. We have found this not to be the case. In fact, one of the reasons for a company to collaborate is to create more publication opportunities for its own scientists and physicians.

We now also see that the patent system levels the playing field in the private sector because patenting the latest technology creates more competitive pressures by making slight but patentable modifications of that technology easier.

As we move into the 1990s, the issue is not the delay of publication but of the patent. The backlog of biotechnology patents at the U.S. Patent and Trademark Office testifies to this point. The issue is not whether to pursue a patent, it is what will happen to the application after it is filed.

Finally, the larger question for a pharmaceutical company is exclusivity, no matter how it is obtained or how it is protected. The best path to exclusivity is innovation, and here again is a primary reason for collaboration with academic medical centers: Exclusivity follows innovation, which follows excellence.

PUBLIC POLICY AS A FACTOR INFLUENCING THE PATTERNS OF ACADEMIC-INDUSTRY COLLABORATION

The primary driving force is technology. A host of new frontiers are on the technological horizon, including, among others: gene therapy, early detection of susceptibles, protein engineering, novel delivery systems (especially for large proteins), receptor technology and design, imaging, diagnostics, oncogenetics, immunomodulation, neurotransmitter regulation, and enzymatic and hormonal control systems.

This technological drive will, in turn, continue to create cost pressures, and research programs will need to achieve all possible economies of scale in order to develop the most cost-effective programs. This is where quality and economy come together—the quality provided by academic medical centers creates added value (and therefore greater economies) in corporate research programs.

The need for personnel will intensify for industry. For instance, right now, there is an ever-increasing demand for physicians with experience in clinical pharmacology. Industry will hire some of these people; others will remain as collaborators/consultants. Aside from clinical pharmacologists, industry will need more and more people who have graduated from or had experience teaching in academic medical centers. These people will range across a wide spectrum of specialties.

Public policy is likely to continue to be economics-driven for at least the next few years. Cost-containment measures and managed-care scenarios will require even better decisions about where one finds the kind of quality one needs in order quickly to develop innovative pharmaceutical products.

The current cost-containment environment is creating a dilemma for research-based industry, which needs to turn out positive quarterly earnings comparisons in order to build shareholder value, but which also needs to invest heavily in the future in order to develop new products. This next-quarter versus next-decade dilemma will continue to be a major determinant of just how many resources individual companies have to invest outside their intramural programs. It has been proposed in some quarters that continued consolidation of the industry is the only way out of this dilemma, but we disagree. We see a continuing place for midsized companies that intensely focus their resources and expertise on those areas to which they are best suited and in which there is the most medical demand.

CONCLUSIONS AND RECOMMENDATIONS

The competitive and financial environments in which the industry finds itself do need to achieve better equilibrium. However, what the pharmaceutical industry needs more than anything else is a stable, vital research base from which to draw new ideas and in which to find new personnel and new collaborations and agreements to fuel its considerable developmental power. We would, therefore, suggest the following:

- Double the NIH budget by 1995.
- Concentrate more on recruiting the "best and brightest" of our own young people into biomedical research.
- Create a private basic-research fund with money coming from products that arise out of collaborative agreements between industry and academia or government.
- Do not subject funding of the basic research enterprise to multiyear budget reconciliations.
- Change the patent system to allow a reasonable period of exclusivity that begins when a pharmaceutical product is first approved for marketing.
- Build on the concepts of the FDA Revitalization Act of 1990, and work with the agency to strengthen it.
- Create many more cross-training programs among industry, the NIH, and academic medical centers.
- Defend the continuing role of tertiary teaching hospitals.

We would like to close this chapter with a statement made by the late A. Bartlett Giamatti when he was president of Yale University: "When we come to cast a retrospective glance on the decade of the eighties, we will find that the universities that acted within an established set of basic principles will still be able to proffer the strengths and quality that attracted industry in the first place" (Langfitt et al. 1983). We could not agree more: Strength and quality are what companies continually seek as complements to their internal programs and as synergistic tools in accomplishing their respective strategic goals.

REFERENCES

Brody, B. 1990. Interview with J. E. Galligan, Public Affairs. Upjohn.

Cooper, T. 1988. *National Institutes of Health STEP Silver Anniversary Forum*. Bethesda, Maryland: National Institutes of Health.

Cooper, T. 1990. Foundations, traditions and directions in U.S. health care. *Vital Speeches of the Day,* 3(17): 79–81.

Langfitt, T., Hackney, S., Fishman, A. P., and Glowasky, A. V. Eds. 1983. *Partners in the Research Enterprise*. Philadelphia: University of Pennsylvania Press, p. 9.

Mahoney, T. 1959. *The Merchants of Life: An Account of the American Pharmaceutical Industry*. Freeport, New York: Books for Libraries Press, pp. 51, 117, 133.

Pinter, D. 1990. Interview with J. E. Galligan, Public Affairs. Upjohn.

Schneiderman, H. 1988. University-Research Partners: The Why's, Do's, and Don'ts. *Conference Board Report: Getting More Out of R&D and Technology,* 904: 45–7.

Sproull, R., Chair. 1984. *Twentieth Century Fund Task Force on the Commercialization of Scientific Research*. New York: Science Business, Priority Press, p. 11.

Varrin, R., and Kukick, D. S. 1985. Guidelines for industry-sponsored research at universities. *Science,* 227: 388.

12 • The National Institutes of Health and Its Interactions with Industry

Philip S. Chen, Jr.

The National Institutes of Health (NIH) had its origin in 1887, when a one-room Laboratory of Hygiene was founded at the Public Health Service (PHS) Marine Hospital, Staten Island, New York (NIH 1991). This was renamed the Hygienic Laboratory in 1891, and moved to Washington, D.C. In 1930, the Hygienic Laboratory was renamed the National Institute of Health, and during this early period, its research efforts were primarily directed toward infectious diseases. However, the NIH was established for the special purpose of pure scientific research, to ascertain the cause, prevention and cure of diseases affecting human beings. Thus, its mission is to uncover new knowledge that will lead to improved health for everyone. NIH works toward that mission by conducting research in its own laboratories; supporting the research of nonfederal scientists in universities, medical schools, hospitals, and research institutions throughout the country and abroad; training research investigators; and fostering and supporting biomedical communication.

Today, the NIH consists of some twenty different institutes, centers, and divisions (ICDs). It is an agency of the PHS, within the U.S. Department of Health and Human Services (DHHS), and is recognized as the focal point for all health research in the United States. The NIH maintains hundreds of laboratories containing complex and highly sophisticated research equipment, a 540-bed research hospital known as the Warren Grant Magnuson Clinical Center, and the National Library of Medicine, the world's largest repository of medical literature and a national center for biomedical communication.

THE NIH INTRAMURAL RESEARCH PROGRAM

The conduct of biomedical research within the walls of NIH is the oldest of the activities of NIH. Twelve of the thirteen institutes have intramural programs, the National Institute of General Medical Sciences being the only exception. In addition, several research centers and divisions, such as the Clinical Center and the National Center for Research Resources, participate in intramural research.

The NIH's intramural programs are generally considered to be of very high caliber, enjoying an international reputation. Some consider them to be the best general medical research institutions in the world. To quote Arthur Kornberg, Professor of Biochemistry at the Stanford University School of Medicine and a Nobel Prize winner, "As for research achievements in the last 25 years, no single institution has so dominated the journals of basic medical science, and some of these contributions have been of stellar magnitude."

Lewis Thomas, a noted medical administrator and author observed that

> the National Institutes of Health is not only the largest institution for biomedical science on earth, it is one of this nation's great treasures. As social inventions for human betterment go, this one is a standing proof that, at least once in a while, government possesses the capacity to do something unique, imaginative, useful, and altogether right. . . . at the center of the NIH scientific effort, driving the whole vast enterprise along, is the so-called Intramural Research Program. Although this represents only a minor portion of the total NIH budget—around 10 percent—for sheer excellence and abundant productivity the institution cannot be matched by any other scientific enterprise anywhere. (Thomas 1984)

THE CONCEPTUAL BASIS OF TECHNOLOGY TRANSFER

In essence, technology transfer is at the heart of the NIH mission. It could be regarded as the way that the practice of medical prevention, diagnosis, or treatment gets changed.

Broadly, it is composed of three components:

1. Publication and oral presentations into the open literature and public domain
2. Consensus development conferences sponsored by the NIH Office of Medical Applications of Research (OMAR), in collaboration with the various institutes

3. Patenting, licensing, and commercial application of research findings into practical items in the armamentarium of the health practitioner or for use by the public

The third, more narrow focus is the formal NIH Technology Transfer Program, for which the Office of Technology Transfer (OTT) is responsible. How has this more narrow focus on Technology Transfer come about? It appears to have arisen, in part, from changes in the culture of biomedical science and its foundation in basic research. This culture was traditionally to disseminate new knowledge freely into the public domain through publications and presentations. Changes in this philosophy have come about for several reasons:

• Recognition that patents and licensing can result in more effective application of research findings into the marketplace
• Rise in the biotechnology industry, in large part due to NIH-supported research advances in molecular biology and recombinant DNA technology
• Relative diminution in the proportion of biomedical research support demands that can be satisfied by U.S. Government Grant and Contract funding, and the consequent need to attract industry financial support or collaboration
• For the U.S. Congress, the desire to see government-produced research (perhaps currently sitting on the shelf) put into commercial application in order to make U.S. industry more competitive in the world marketplace

THE STEVENSON-WYDLER TECHNOLOGY INNOVATION ACT OF 1980

Public Law 96-480 (Stevenson-Wydler Technology Innovation Act of 1980) was signed by President Carter on October 21, 1980. Its purpose was "to promote United States technological innovation for the achievement of national economic, environmental, and social goals, and for other purposes."

The Stevenson-Wydler Act was based on two U.S. Congressional perceptions:

1. Technology and industrial innovation are central to the economic, environmental, and social well-being of citizens of the United States.
2. Technology and industrial innovation offer an improved standard of living, increased public and private sector productivity, creation of

new industries and employment opportunities, improved public services, and enhanced competitiveness of U.S. products in world markets.

Congress further noted that "many new discoveries and advances in science occur in universities and federal laboratories, while the application of this new knowledge to commercial and useful public purposes depends largely upon actions by business and labor. Cooperation among academia, federal laboratories, labor, and industry, in such forms as technology transfer, personnel exchange, joint research projects and others, should be renewed, expanded, and strengthened," and that, "small businesses have performed an important role in advancing industrial and technological innovation."

It was felt that there was a need for "a comprehensive national policy—to enhance technological innovation for commercial and public purposes—including a strong national policy supporting domestic technology transfer and utilization of the science and technology resources of the federal government."

The Stevenson-Wydler Act authorized the Department of Commerce (DOC) and The National Science Foundation (NSF) to establish Centers for Industrial Technology—nonprofit institutions to be affiliated with universities or other nonprofit organizations intended to foster participation of individuals from industry and universities in cooperative technological innovation activities.

To support technology transfer, the act required that after September 30, 1981, each agency with federal laboratories allocate at least 0.5 percent of the agency's research and development budget for this purpose, and that each federal laboratory having a total annual budget exceeding $20,000,000 provide at least one full-time professional position as staff for its Office of Research and Technology Applications (ORTA). At the NIH, the OMAR was designated as its ORTA, until the Office of Technology Transfer was created after passage of the Federal Technology Transfer Act of 1986.

BARRIERS CREATED BY PRIOR FEDERAL PATENT POLICIES

Despite the passage of the Stevenson-Wydler Act, some agency officials believed that existing federal patent/licensing policies were barriers to transferring federally developed technologies to the marketplace. Approximately 15 percent of the respondents to a General Accounting Office (GAO) questionnaire indicated that patent/licensing restrictions inhibited the transfer of federally owned technologies because of the uncertainty of receiving a patent, title, or exclusive license. Also, the complexities of the process of securing a title or license deterred firms from investing in federally owned technologies. Some agency officials noted that without exclusive licenses, firms may not invest in federally owned technologies.

THE BAYH-DOLE ACT

In December 1980, President Carter signed the Patent and Trademark Laws Amendment of 1980 (Public Law 96-517, also known as the Bayh-Dole Act), which gives first preference in the exclusive or partially exclusive licensing of federally owned inventions to nonprofit organizations and small business firms. In February 1983, President Reagan issued a directive to agencies to make the provisions of Public Law 96-517 applicable to all (i.e., including large businesses) contractors. This directive was intended to provide an incentive for private industry to commercialize inventions developed with federal funds.

The Bayh-Dole Act is applicable to extramural organizations supported by government grants or contracts, which, for the NIH, is fully 80 percent of the total budget, currently (fiscal year [FY] 1991) around $8 billion. The Bayh-Dole Act allows the awardee to take ownership of intellectual property rights to discoveries made under government support, and thus to patent, license, collect, and retain royalties, and so on, as long as the royalties are shared, in part, with the inventor and the remainder used for scientific research or education purposes. As a result of the Bayh-Dole Act, many universities are setting up licensing offices, and the new profession of university technology development promoters has blossomed.

THE FEDERAL TECHNOLOGY TRANSFER ACT OF 1986 (FTTA)

The FTTA builds on and extends the principles enunciated in the Stevenson-Wydler Act of 1980 and the Bayh-Dole Act of 1980, to stimulate the transfer of government laboratory-developed technology into commercial application. Incentives are offered for companies and federal laboratories to enter into cooperative research and development agreements (CRADAs), which spell out the terms of collaborative research efforts. The U.S. Congressional intent in passing the FTTA was further to stimulate the commercialization of research results from federal laboratories. Patented inventions developed under a CRADA can be licensed exclusively to the participating company, with the resulting license fees and royalties being shared with the government inventor and the remainder being retained by the laboratory for technology transfer purposes.

The act authorizes the government to commit resources such as personnel, equipment, and material—but not funds—to a collaborator and to accept similar resources, including outside funds, in the conduct of specified research projects.

Implementation of the FTTA by the PHS reflects five general principles: (1) awareness of its dual mission relating to basic biomedical research as well as serving a regulatory role, (2) adoption of procedures that complement but do not unduly complicate research efforts, (3) recognition that public health and U.S. industrial competitiveness both are served by efficient technology transfer activities, (4) decentralized technology transfer authority, and (5) the involvement of industry in the review of emerging guidelines and draft model agreements.

Under the auspices of the FTTA, the PHS agencies have entered into about 115 active CRADAs, of which more than one fourth are with small businesses. These CRADAs vary widely in their research projects and include the development of AIDS therapeutics, diagnostic test kits for cancer and infectious diseases, transgenic animals, genetic therapy, and various types of bio-instrumentation.

THE DHHS TECHNOLOGY TRANSFER STRUCTURE

Because the federal laboratories within the DHHS are components of the PHS, the Office of the Assistant Secretary for Health (OASH) assumed an early role in FTTA implementation. Several meetings were convened by the Deputy Assistant Secretary for Health of a Technology Management Advisory Board (TMAB), consisting of the deputy directors of each of the involved agencies, plus the principal technology transfer official of each agency.

Within the DHHS, the principal federal laboratory involved in technology transfer is the National Institutes of Health. The NIH director appointed a Patent Policy Board chaired by the Associate Director for Intramural Affairs. The board sets overall policies and has developed an operational structure to oversee FTTA implementation. The Alcohol, Drug Abuse and Mental Health Administration (ADAMHA), and the Centers for Disease Control (CDC) joined the Patent Policy Board as full partners. Liaison members from the Food and Drug Administration (FDA), the OASH, and the Department of Commerce's National Technical Information Service (NTIS) attend monthly meetings of the board. Working subcommittees of the Patent Policy Board have been established, with responsibility for cooperative research and development agreements, royalty distribution, data systems, training, the annual PHS Collaboration Forum, and the technology development coordinators (TDC).

The DHHS Technology Transfer Program has received recognition as being a leader among government agencies (e.g., by the chairman of the Executive Working Group of the Interagency Committee for Federal Laboratory Technology Transfer at the Department of Commerce, which coordinates FTTA implementation governmentwide). Testimony presented before several subcommittees of Congress has also described the DHHS implementation program as exemplary among government agencies (Adler 1989, 1991; Chen 1989a, 1989b, 1990a, 1990b).

THE OFFICE OF TECHNOLOGY TRANSFER (OTT)

The principal new organizational component is the OTT, located within the NIH Office of Intramural Affairs. Office of the Director. (Established in 1988, it was originally named the Office of Invention Development [OID].)

The patent branch, earlier a part of the Office of General Counsel, DHHS, is now a component of the OTT. It is responsible for processing invention reports from intramural scientists and for obtaining patent protection in the United States. Currently, much of the actual patent prosecution work is still carried out under contract with outside law firms.

A number of activities of the Patent Policy Board and the OTT are of interest:

- Development of a policy statement that presents the NIH/ADAMHA basic research and collaboration philosophy
- Development of a model CRADA, which has greatly facilitated negotiations leading to collaborative projects
- Development of a model Materials Transfer Agreement
- Initiation of the Annual Public Health Service Technology Transfer Forums, bringing together government and industry representatives and assuring "equal access"; an associated directory is published annually
- Convening of a Retreat on Conflict of Interest in Collaborations with Industry
- Drafting of Model Patent License Agreements

- Implementation, thus far, of well over 100 CRADAs
- Preparation of the Technology Transfer Workbook and conducting of semiannual briefing sessions for all concerned NIH/ADAMHA scientists and administrative staff
- Establishment of a system of TDCs, who comprise a network of implementing staff within each NIH/ADAMHA component
- Scheduling of regular Technology Transfer Grand Round Meetings (including outside speakers)
- Convening of Technology Management Team Meetings (to develop licensing strategies for each invention on a case-by-case basis)

IMPORTANT ISSUES

The Patent Policy Board and its various subcommittees continue to address a number of important issues that are of concern in FTTA implementation. New issues arise periodically. The issues are both legal and policy in nature; some will require extensive discussion and/or higher-level guidance to resolve. Among the issues that concern the DHHS are

- Protection, and royalty sharing, for government developers of computer software (government employees currently may not copyright)
- Pricing of products developed with federal support
- Whether extramural scientists should be allowed to enter into CRADAs
- Whether extramural grant or contract funds can be used by an outside organization toward a CRADA
- To what extent a scientist collaborating under a CRADA can later be allowed to consult for a company that may obtain a license to a CRADA-developed invention

PHILOSOPHICAL DIFFERENCE BETWEEN ACADEMIC INSTITUTIONS AND NIH WITH REGARD TO COLLABORATIONS WITH INDUSTRY

A significant philosophical aspect pertaining to the NIH that may not be as germane to many other government laboratories is the closeness with which it associates itself, culturally, to the academic world. NIH scientific staff, though they be government employees, are regarded much like medical school faculty. Indeed, the NIH was the postdoctoral research training ground for many of the current leaders in academic medicine today. This fortuitous circumstance came to pass because during the Korean and Vietnam Wars, young physicians and other doctorates could serve their military draft obligation by serving as PHS Commissioned Officers in the NIH intramural laboratories and clinics. The ability to learn and to perform full-time biomedical research for a period of several years allowed many of these bright young physicians and Ph.D.s to leapfrog over their contemporaries on the outside by a process that has been called the "NIH shunt."

Today, hundreds of young doctorate-level scientists spend varying periods of time in research training at the NIH; Ph.D. candidates perform their thesis research here; and medical students take a year out in the Howard Hughes Medical Institute–NIH Research Scholars Program. There are also medical students who take two-month clinical elective courses, and high school and college students who work during the school year or summers to gain science experience and to earn money toward their education. The geographic location of NIH in Bethesda, Maryland, is popularly known as the NIH "campus." Historically, the NIH scientific staff came from the academic world, and that is where they tended to go if they left the NIH. They are encouraged to perform scholarly activities, such as editing, writing, giving lectures in the Foundation for Advanced Education in the Sciences (FAES) evening school, organizing and conducting workshops, seminars, and symposia, and publishing extensively in the open literature. Thus, the NIH scientific staff are regarded as the moral equivalent of university faculty, and within the constraints of government laws and regulations, an attempt is made to treat them as such.

CONSULTING FOR INDUSTRY

In contrast with official collaborative relationships between NIH scientists and industry, there are other types of contacts performed as approved "outside work" on the scientist's own time and outside of official duty. Before August 1980, such outside work for industry was not permitted under the NIH rules. At that time, NIH policy was modified to permit intramural scientists to give lectures of an open nature to industry for an honorarium, subject to the existing rules. The basic rationale was that such open material was already in the public domain and that, therefore, anyone should have the right to speak about it.

James Wyngaarden, who became the director of NIH on April 30, 1982, heard from some senior NIH scientists that changing circumstances made it desirable to reexamine the long-standing policy that prohibited consulting by NIH staff. The two major problems appeared to be the increasing disparity between the income of NIH scientists and that of comparable scientists on the outside, and the inability of NIH scientists to interact closely with, or participate in, the new biotechnology developments occurring in industry, factors either or both of which might induce NIH staff to leave for the more lucrative academic or industrial sectors.

Another advantage for academic faculty is related to possible income from inventions. The Bayh-Dole Act gave ownership of inventions made by government extramural grantees or contractors to the nonprofit institution or small business, and a faculty inventor would receive a share of the royalty stream. University faculty were thus becoming increasingly involved in consulting for, and even in the management of, new biotechnology companies. I was appointed by the NIH Director to chair a committee on outside work, to examine the consulting issue, along with several other outside work issues, such as what should be permissible activity for high-level officials, for clinical practice, and for extramural administrators. Based on the recommendations of the committee, Wyngaarden promulgated a new policy, published as the NIH Manual Chapter 2300-735-4 on "Outside Work and Activities," dated August 1, 1985. The most recent revision was issued September 1, 1988.

The major change was that, subject to a variety of restrictions and safeguards, NIH scientists would be permitted to consult, on their own time, for profit-making companies so long as no government information not already in the public domain (that is, published or presented at an open meeting) was given to the company as a result of the paid consultation. In other words, the consultations could be based on the NIH scientist's general expertise in an area, but not on information relating to current research in the scientist's laboratory. A number of restrictions were then imposed or have been added, as a result of experience. The maximum amount that could be received from one company per year was $12,500, with an overall annual maximum of $25,000. The scientist had to perform the consultation while on annual leave or during weekends or in the evenings. The scientist was not allowed to own stock or to receive stock options in the company for which he or she consulted, and service on a board of directors was not permitted, although the scientist could serve on a scientific advisory committee or its equivalent, provided that not more than one third of the members were from the NIH. This was to avoid having companies that looked like NIH spin-offs with favored access to NIH intramural research technology.

CONFLICT OF INTEREST CONSIDERATIONS RAISED BY THE FTTA

With the enactment of the FTTA of 1986, various questions arose regarding the applicability of existing conflict of interest statutes and regulations to the activities of federal inventors under the act. The emphasis that the FTTA placed on invention disclosure, patenting, and licensing necessitated examination of whether additional restrictions were needed to prevent conflicts and improprieties from arising in the course of implementation of the FTTA.

The following is a summary of relevant statutes and regulations that comprise the ethical framework applicable to federal employees. These relate both to criminal prohibitions and to standards of conduct.

Criminal Prohibitions

Financial interests—self-dealing: 18 U.S.C. 208 prohibits employees from participating in an official capacity in any matter in which they, members of their immediate family, or an organization with which they are associated have a financial interest.

Representational activities before the government: 18 U.S.C. 203 and 205 prohibit an employee from receiving any compensation for services rendered and from acting in a representational capacity for an individual or organization outside the federal government in connection with its dealings with the government.

Augmentation of salary: 18 U.S.C. 209 prohibits employees from accepting anything from a source other than the U.S. government as compensation for the performance of their duties.

Postemployment restrictions: 18 U.S.C. 207 prohibits employees from engaging in certain activities relating to their former agency or duties on behalf of parties outside the government after leaving government service.

Standards of Conduct

Under Executive Order 11222, the DHHS has issued Standards of Conduct applicable to all its employees. These standards set forth rules relating to the avoidance of appearances of conflicts of interest; limitations on outside employment and other outside activities; prohibitions on the acceptance of gifts from entities doing business with the department, regulated entities, and others with interests that might be affected by the performance of an employee's duties; and certain other standards relating to behavior on the job. In general, the standards admonish employees against using their public office for private gain, giving preferential treatment, impeding government efficiency or economy, or taking other actions that may adversely affect the confidence of the public in the integrity of the government. Some DHHS components have issued supplements to these standards, which apply specifically to their employees (e.g., the NIH Manual Chapter 2300-735-4 on "Outside Work and Activities," NIH 1988).

POTENTIAL CONFLICT SITUATIONS UNDER FTTA

Some of the possible conflict of interest or standards of conduct questions that might arise fall into several categories:

1. Conflicts that may arise in the development of collaborations
2. Disclosure of collaborations and other arrangements
3. Participation by employee inventors in decisions on licensing and collaborations
4. Postemployment restrictions

Conflicts that May Arise in the Development of Collaborations

Where employees have consulting arrangements or are otherwise employed by outside companies, where they own stock or a partnership interest in such a company, or where they have recently been employed by that company, there can be a real or apparent conflict of interest in those employees being involved in a collaborative agreement to do joint research with that company in their official capacities. (NIH internal regulations prohibit the approval of a request for an employee to do outside consulting for a firm with which the scientist's laboratory is collaborating.) Conflict of interest guidelines being followed by the NIH include the following:

- Employees may not participate in any collaboration with an outside company with which they are employed in a consulting or other capacity.
- Employees may not participate in any collaboration with an outside company in which they or a member of their immediate family has a financial interest.
- Employees must disclose to the agency any negotiations or arrangements for future employment they enter into with a collaborating party so that the agency can assess the propriety and extent of their continued participation in the collaboration.

- An additional question may arise with respect to the holding of financial interests or outside positions with organizations that enter into a CRADA with a particular laboratory, but where the employee holding those interests is not directly involved in the CRADA. These situations may present appearance problems and probably should be avoided.
- Employees should not use any information that comes into their possession in the course of their scientific research or otherwise (i.e., insider information) for their own or anyone else's personal gain.

Each proposed CRADA includes a form entitled "Conflict of Interest and Fair Access Survey," in which the NIH/ADAMHA Principal Investigator certifies with respect to the following:

1. (Absence of) financial interest on the part of the principal investigator, spouse, or minor children "in any interest of monetary value which may be predictably affected by the official action of the employee." Normally, "financial interest" includes salaries, stocks, or consultant agreements, but not royalties from inventions licensed by the government. (The Office of Government Ethics in a September 28, 1988, letter to the Department of Commerce concluded that federal inventors' interest in whatever royalty share may be paid to them under the Technology Transfer Act should not be considered a financial interest as that term is used in 18 U.S.C. 208.) In special cases, a waiver of the financial interest can be approved by the institute after consultation with the Office of General Counsel, DHHS.
2. (Absence of) outside work activities with the proposed collaborator.
3. (Justification for) selection of a collaborator includes information about when negotiations began, any other CRADAs with the proposed collaborator, and why the particular proposed collaborator was selected, such as unique technology, expertise, materials/equipment, or facilities. Information is also to be provided about how the proposed collaborator learned of the opportunity to collaborate on the project, such as through the PHS Technology Transfer Forum, the PHS Technology Transfer Directory, or advertisement in the *Federal Register.*

Disclosure of Collaborations and Other Arrangements

The potential exists for employees to begin collaborative ventures with outside organizations and to make private deals with such organizations with respect to inventions arising under the collaboration before any formal agreement is entered into between the agency and the organization. In order to avoid prejudice to the government's rights in any such collaboration, prompt disclosure and approval by superior levels of administration are required of all scientists.

Participation by Employee Inventors in Decisions on Licensing and Collaborations

Where an employee has patentable ideas, has reported an invention for possible patenting, or is named on a patent being considered for licensing, questions may be raised about the appropriateness of his or her participating in decisions regarding collaborations or licensing. Such decisions may have an impact on royalties ultimately received by the agency and the inventor. Yet the best individual to advise the agency on the desirability of particular collaborative arrangements or particular companies with which to collaborate may well be the inventor. The Technology Management Team approach allows the inventor to contribute appropriate inputs into the licensing consideration process, but distances the inventor from the final decision making. Participation in the following activities may sometimes be necessary or appropriate but should be limited by careful supervision and approval by officials senior to the inventor:

- Clinical trials relating to the invention
- FDA review of the invention under an investigational new drug (IND) exemption or new drug application (NDA).
- Agency general policymaking regarding development and use of the invention
- Decisions regarding granting, modifying, or terminating of license agreements
- Decisions of the agency regarding the development or approval of improvement or replacement technology

Postemployment Restrictions

An employee who has participated in a collaborative agreement or has been named as an inventor on an agency invention and who leaves the agency is under specific restrictions relating to the subject matter of the collaboration or the invention. While not prohibited from continuing to work on the invention for another entity, he or she may not, under 18 U.S.C. 207(a) represent anyone before any federal agency with respect to that subject. For example, if an NIH inventor leaves the agency and goes to work for a pharmaceutical firm, he or she may not represent the firm in its dealings with FDA over the subject matter of that invention or the subject matter of a collaborative effort in which he or she was involved. He or she may, however, assist the firm behind the scenes in the preparation of materials and arguments with respect to the invention.

OUTREACH ACTIVITIES OF THE NIH TECHNOLOGY TRANSFER PROGRAM

Informing and advising commercial firms about opportunities to collaborate with PHS scientists is a key responsibility of the OTT. The OTT welcomes the opportunity both to discuss technology transfer from PHS agencies with companies and to add company profiles and contact persons to the OTT database of potential CRADA partners and licensees. Such outreach efforts are designed to augment the customary contacts made by PHS scientists with their private-sector colleagues arising from publication in professional journals or interactions at professional society meetings.

All of the ICDs of NIH, ADAMHA, CDC, and the FDA have at least one person responsible for coordinating technology transfer matters, particularly CRADAs. These individuals, known as TDCs, are often the best source for information about specific areas of research projects. To contact a TDC directly, interested parties can obtain the names and phone numbers from the OTT.

Office of Technology Transfer
Control Data Building, Room 310P
6003 Executive Boulevard
Rockville, MD 20852
Tel. (301) 496-3561
FAX: (301) 402-0220

The OTT also has a special outreach program that strives to involve small businesses across the country in collaborative opportunities, through communications with state and local technology development organizations.

Conferences

In addition to periodic seminars and briefings, two major conferences a year are sponsored by the OTT, bringing together hundreds of representatives from industry, government, and academia to communicate regarding common interests in technology transfer. In the spring, the OTT cosponsors (with the Pharmaceutical Manufacturers Association) a technology transfer policy conference, the first of which was held March 1–2, 1990, at the Georgetown University Conference Center.

Each fall, the OTT sponsors the PHS Technology Transfer Forum, intended to bring government and private-sector scientists together to discuss research areas of mutual interests. Initiated in 1988, the first two forums were one-day meetings commencing with plenary talks, followed by poster session presentations of current research by PHS scientists to company representatives. The format has now changed into a more focused topical format, with the third forum on November 8–9, 1990, addressed to Transgenic Animals Research (first day) and Central Nervous System Drug Development (second day). New topics are covered each year. A major purpose of the forums is to ensure that all interested companies have the opportunity to learn about opportunities for CRADA collaboration with PHS scientists.

Electronic Bulletin Board

The OTT has recently created an electronic bulletin board, which contains a variety of essential technology transfer data. This service, PHS-OTTO (Office of Technology Transfer On-line) [301-496-0750] can be accessed via modem 24 hours a day. PHS-OTTO contains downloadable copies of PHS technology transfer guidelines and model agreements, a list of current CRADAs and participating PHS scientists, summaries of inventions available for licensing, and downloadable full-text files of patent applications available for licensing.

Publications

An OTT information packet about CRADAs and other matters related to technology transfer from PHS agencies is available from the OTT, upon request, along with a comprehensive PHS Technology Transfer Director that provides a hard copy of information found in PHS-OTTO, including model Material Transfer Agreements and model License Agreements.

THE CRADA

Under the FTTA of 1986, Congress encouraged the utilization of CRADAs to enhance and facilitate collaboration between governmental agencies and commercial firms. The FTTA provides the authority and an effective mechanism to enter into joint research and development (R&D) projects.

Under a CRADA with the PHS, a joint research project is specified, along with the respective contributions of the government and collaborator. The PHS agency provides research personnel, laboratory facilities, materials, equipment, supplies, and other in-kind contributions—but not funding—to the collaborator. In general, the collaborator contributes personnel, equipment, and materials. The collaborator also may contribute funds to cover some of the added costs to the participating agency for work done under the research program of the agreement. Ultimately, the collaborator is responsible for commercialization of a new product, process, or service.

The primary difference between CRADAs and other PHS research contracts and agreements is that CRADAs provide the commercial collaborator with an option in advance to negotiate exclusive licenses to inventions made under the agreement. Also, in carrying out the scope of work specified in the CRADA, PHS scientists are encouraged to work closely with private firms to investigate and develop technology jointly, based on the scientists' research interests.

As with other collaborative agreements, the PHS agency enters into a CRADA only when the research objective is consistent with the agency's mission. Because PHS CRADAs do not seek sponsorship, but rather collaboration, CRADAs are a very cost-effective way for companies, particularly small businesses, to leverage their own R&D efforts.

A typical CRADA between a PHS agency and a commercial firm includes a number of standard provisions, based on policy guidelines and model agreements adopted by the PHS agencies. These include

- Research, development, and commercialization efforts contemplated for each party
- Contributions of the PHS agency by way of equipment, supplies, and personnel
- Contributions of the commercial firm by way of equipment, supplies, personnel, and funding
- Confidentiality
- Publication of results
- Inventions, focusing on definitions, ownership, and patent prosecution
- Licensing
- Liability

The Benefits of CRADAs?

Collaboration under a CRADA results in a number of mutual benefits for PHS agencies and commercial firms, and it expedites public access to technology developments. Commercial firms benefit by

- Improved access to PHS scientists and facilities
- Better access to expertise related to research results and inventions
- Options to exclusive licenses on inventions made under the agreement
- Profitable new products and processes

PHS agencies benefit by

- Improved access to industry scientists and facilities
- Accelerated interaction with industry to transfer basic research findings to the commercial development process
- Increased familiarity with problems related to commercialization of products and processes
- Sharing of royalty income for both individual inventors and PHS agencies

Training

The training and education of scientists and support staff about technology transfer and collaborative opportunities with industry are other key elements of the OTT program. To this end, semiannual training seminars are held to explain the rudiments of CRADAs, patents, and patent licensing agreements to the PHS scientific community. A comprehensive training notebook prepared by the OTT also is distributed widely throughout the PHS.

The OTT also sponsors "Technology Transfer Grand Rounds," a monthly speaker series where guest lecturers from industry, venture capital organizations, and the patent bar, among others, interact with PHS scientists. Additional in-house training initiatives include periodic "Technology Transfer Briefings."

Patent Prosecution

Obtaining patents is a key component of PHS technology transfer activities because patents allow full public disclosure while laying a foundation for business development. Patents facilitate rapid commercialization of an invention through licensing agreements with commercial firms.

Since passage of the FTTA, major agencies within the PHS have stepped up their efforts to seek patents for the work of government inventors. Seeking patents is a critical step in protecting the rights of PHS agencies and individual inventors who share royalties through commercialization of their research efforts.

THE MANAGEMENT OF TECHNOLOGY

The OTT technology management program primarily focuses on matching research with potential commercial collaborators or licensees. This is done through review and evaluation of the technology portfolio of NIH, ADAMHA, and CDC, as well as through monitoring of the scientific and business literature to identify and approach companies likely to have a licensing or collaboration interest.

The central component of the OTT technology management process is the technology management team (TMT) meeting, which reviews the licensing potential of newly filed patent applications on a case-by-case basis. Attending these meetings are inventors and representatives from their respective institutes, along with technology management, patent, and licensing specialists from the OTT.

At the TMT meeting, an attempt is made to identify all related patent applications in the PHS, so that interrelated technology can be licensed in a commercially useful package. Additionally, the team discusses the potential for separately licensing a given package of technology to several companies that will develop products for different fields of use, such as diagnostics, instrumentation, and therapeutics.

The OTT is compiling a database that will enable OTT staff to identify the persons responsible for business and product development or licensing at pharmaceutical, biotechnology, and other companies that are potential licensees or collaborators. All companies are invited to participate in the database by submitting information about licensing interests and designating contact personnel.

TECHNOLOGY LICENSING

The purposes of the technology licensing program for the PHS agencies are to transfer the result of laboratory research, to benefit public health through commercial applications, and to stimulate further research by sharing royalty income with inventors and laboratories.

In carrying out the licensing function of technology transfer, the OTT directly handles licensing of inventions made under CRADAs.

Licensing negotiations are carried out using, as a starting point, a model licensing agreement drafted by the OTT. The OTT also facilitates and oversees licensing activities carried out by the NTIS of the DOC, which acts as the PHS licensing agent in many cases. In FY 1990, 48 licenses were granted, and a similar number are expected in FY 1991. Since 1977, over 340 license agreements have been executed on behalf of PHS agencies, the majority from the NIH.

Technology Licensing Objectives

The following types of licenses are available:

1. Patent licenses
   a. nonexclusive
   b. exclusive
2. Commercial Evaluation Licenses
3. Biological Material Licenses (for use of nonpatented materials)

The OTT has developed a model patent license agreement that serves as the basis for technology transfer. Its terms and requirements reflect general industry practices and are similar to license agreements used in academia. Some provisions are required by federal law, such as the domestic production of products to be sold in the United States. Federal law also requires public notice through the *Federal Register* when an intramural invention is exclusively licensed.

A business development plan, submitted as part of the license application, serves as the basis for establishing performance benchmarks that are included in the license agreement. The OTT works closely with licensees to monitor performance and to adjust benchmarks when appropriate, to ensure successful commercial development of PHS inventions.

As a result of their comprehensive research programs, PHS agencies frequently seek both domestic and foreign patents on research related to health care products, processes, and services. These patent applications and issued patents serve as the basis for licensing arrangements with private-sector firms and thus encourage and facilitate commercial development of new health care products.

The OTT technology licensing program implements, on behalf of the PHS, various statutes that authorize government agencies to grant patent licenses. These statutes include the Stevenson-Wydler and Bayh-Dole Acts, now codified with federal patent law in Title 35 of the U.S. Code. Regulations governing patent licenses are published in Title 37 of the Code of Federal Regulations, Part 404. License fees and royalties are negotiable, reflecting the rates conventionally requested by academia for inventions with similar commercial potential at about the same stage of development.

For government-owned patents that are not the result of collaborative research under a CRADA, government regulations reflect a preference for nonexclusive licenses. Exclusive licenses are available, however, when appropriate to promote successful commercial development of an invention. Criteria for exclusive license applications include evaluation of whether

- Exclusive licensing serves the best interests of the public
- Practical application of the invention is not likely to be achieved under a nonexclusive license
- An exclusive or partially exclusive license is a reasonable and necessary incentive to promote the investment of risk capital to bring the invention to practical application
- Exclusive license terms and conditions are not broader than necessary
- Exclusive licensing will not lessen competition

Applicants seeking an exclusive license are required to submit a detailed justification of these criteria. Notice of each proposed exclusive license must be published in the *Federal Register,* to provide opportunity for a sixty-day public comment period. The latter requirement is a primary reason why the FTTA is stimulating collaborations between government scientists and industry because CRADA-derived patents may be licensed exclusively to a company without going through such an onerous process.

Commercial firms interested in licensing technology from PHS agencies should contact the OTT for information on licensing opportunities and procedures. The OTT maintains a centralized database of PHS agency inventions available for licensing. In those cases for which the DOC has been given custody of a patent for licensing, the OTT refers the interested party to the appropriate licensing specialist at NTIS.

Information about potential license opportunities also is available from PHS-OTTO. As mentioned previously, PHS-OTTO contains summaries of inventions available for licensing, as well as a list of current CRADAs, CRADA opportunities, participating PHS scientists, and downloadable full-text files of model license agreements and other technology transfer information. OTT also furnishes a printed information packet to interested parties, including the comprehensive *PHS Technology Transfer Directory.* In addition, patents and patent applications from all government agencies are published periodically in the *Federal Register* and in the *Official Gazette of the U.S. Patent and*

Trademark Office. Both documents are available through the U.S. Government Printing Office and through many libraries.

Information on patents and patent applications from all government agencies, including PHS agencies, also is contained in *Government Inventions for Licensing*, a weekly publication of the NTIS. Inventions that may have a greater commercial potential are highlighted in this publication, which is available on an annual subscription basis.

CONCLUSION

The FTTA provides a powerful mechanism for harnessing commercial development to basic research efforts. Collaboration is very much a two-way street; experience to date shows the benefits to the NIH's own research agenda of access to corporate facilities and scientists. In implementing the FTTA, however, a major worry is that conflicts of interest, driven by greed, could warp the biomedical research culture and research agenda of the NIH/ADAMHA. The policies and processes that are developed within the DHHS by the Patent Policy Board must continually strive to minimize that possibility. Public confidence in the integrity and objectivity of DHHS Intramural Research must be preserved; therefore, the magnitude and scope of the Technology Transfer Program must be considered with care and should be appropriate to the overall mission of the agency.

Today, we stand on the threshold of a new era in government-industry relationships, both with respect to basic research, and to development and commercialization. The challenge for government is to be able wisely to conceptualize and implement policies and practices that will avoid the many pitfalls that will beset the unwary. The motivations of the kinds of scientists that the NIH and ADAMHA wish to keep, or hope to attract, must not be so altered by the possibility of royalty dollars as an end that the institution itself will be weakened, either in fact or in the eyes of the public, upon whose trust and financial resources they depend. The goals of the NIH now include improving the economic health of industry and the nation, as well as the physical and mental health of the American public.

REFERENCES

Adler, R. 1989. U.S. Congress, House Committee on Science, Space, and Technology; Subcommittee on Science, Research, and Technology. *Imple-*

mentation of the Federal Technology Transfer Act: Hearing, 101st Congress, 1st sess., 1 June, pp. 170–226.

Adler, R. 1991. U.S. Congress, House Committee on Science, Space, and Technology; Subcommittee on Technology and Competitiveness. *Transfer of Technology from Federal Laboratories: Hearing*, 102d Congress, 1st sess., 30 May, pp. 153–69.

Chen, P. S. 1989. U.S. Congress, House Committee on the Judiciary; Subcommittee on Courts, Intellectual Property, and the Administration of Justice. *Transgenic Animal Patent Reform Act of 1989: Hearing on H.R. 1556*, 101st Congress, 1st sess., 13, 14 September, pp. 154–64.

Chen, P. S. 1989. U.S. Congress, House Committee on Small Business; Subcommittee on Regulation, Business Opportunities, and Energy. *Obstacles to Technology Transfer and Commercialization at Federal Laboratories: Hearing*, 101st Congress, 1st sess., 5 October, pp. 58–65, 185–210.

Chen, P. S. 1990. U.S. Congress, Senate Committee on Small Business. *Technology Transfer and Small Business: Hearing*, 101st Congress, 2nd sess., 8 March, pp. 88–115.

Chen, P. S. 1990. U.S. Congress, House Committee on Science, Space, and Technology; Subcommittee on Science, Research, and Technology. *Transfer of Technology from the Federal Laboratories: Hearing*, 101st Congress, 2nd sess., 3 May, pp. 172–85.

National Institutes of Health. 1988. Manual 2300-735-4. Outside Work and Activities. 1 September.

NIH Almanac 1991. National Institutes of Health Publication No. 91-5. April, p. 142.

Thomas, L. 1984. Foreword. In Stetten, D., and Carrigan, W. T., eds., *NIH: An Account of Research in its Laboratories and Clinics*. Orlando, Florida: Academic Press.

Index

AAMC. *See* Association of American Medical Colleges
AAU. *See* Association of American Universities
AAUP. *See* American Association of University Professors
Academic-industry interactions: biomedical science's needs and approaches to research, 93–95; critical elements in collaboration, 100–105; customization of collaborative agreements, 194–95; development of relationships, 48–51; examples of relationships, 105–17; federal legislation and, 99–100; history of, 188–91; public policy and, 196–97; research patterns, 95–99; "science for sale," 27–31. *See also* Conflicts of interest; Ethical considerations
Academic research: before 1975, 96–97; after 1975, 98–99; animal research, 20–23. *See also* Research and development
ACE. *See* American Council on Education
Acquired immunodeficiency syndrome, 15, 60, 194, 204; HIV, 13, 14
ADAMHA. *See* Alcohol, Drug Abuse, and Mental Health Administration
Adverse publicity, 89–90

AHC. *See* Association of Academic Health Centers
AIDS. *See* Acquired immunodeficiency syndrome
Alcohol, Drug Abuse, and Mental Health Administration, 40, 41, 167–68, 204. *See also* Public Health Service
AMA. *See* American Medical Association
American Association of University Professors, 169, 171, 173
American Council on Education, 169, 171
American Federation for Clinical Research, 130, 142, 147
American Medical Association, 127, 139, 159, 169
Anesthesia, 10
Animal research, 20–23
"Are Scientific Misconduct and Conflicts of Interest Hazardous to Our Health," 84
"Assessing Medical Technologies," 24
Association of Academic Health Centers, 169–70, 171
Association of American Medical Colleges, 170, 171, 176
Association of American Universities, 169